THE VEGAN KETOGENIC DIET COOKBOOK

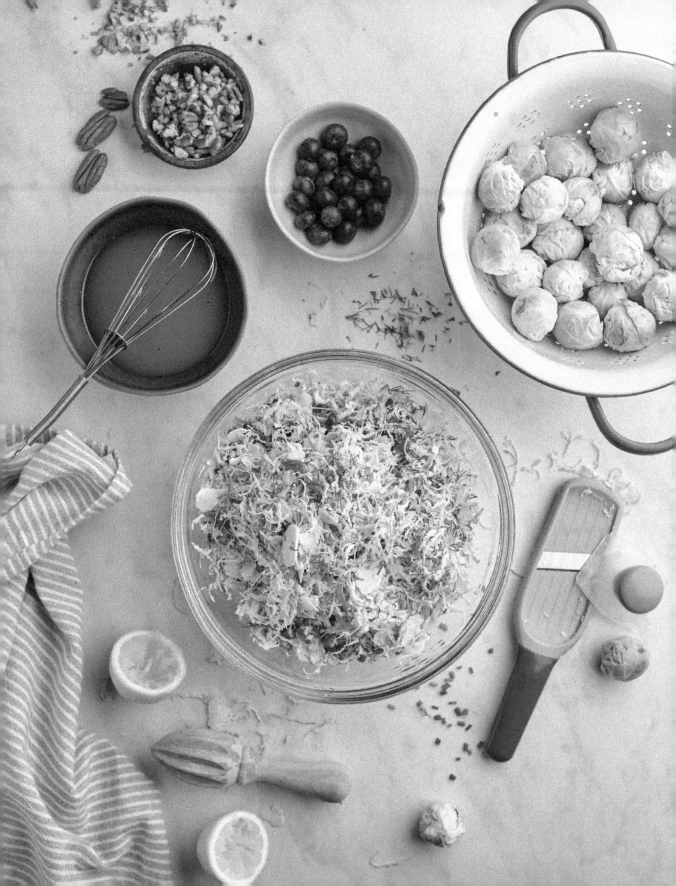

— THE —
VEGAN
KETOGENIC DIET
— COOKBOOK —

75 SATISFYING HIGH-FAT, LOW-CARB, DAIRY-FREE RECIPES

NICOLE DERSEWEH | WHITNEY LAURITSEN

PHOTOGRAPHY BY DARREN MUIR

ROCKRIDGE
PRESS

For general information on our other products and services or to obtain technical support, please contact our Customer Care Department within the United States at (866) 744-2665, or outside the United States at (510) 253-0500.

Rockridge Press publishes its books in a variety of electronic and print formats. Some content that appears in print may not be available in electronic books, and vice versa.

Interior and Cover Designer: Eric Pratt
Art Producer: Karen Williams
Editor: Carolyn Abate
Production Editor: Mia Moran
Photography © 2019 Darren Muir. Food styling by Darren Muir.
Author photos courtesy of © Yoko Morimoto

ISBN: Print 978-1-64152-653-1| eBook 978-1-64152-654-8

R1

For anyone on a mission to bring more love, acceptance, and peace into the world. It all starts with you. We hope this book enriches your body, mind, and heart.

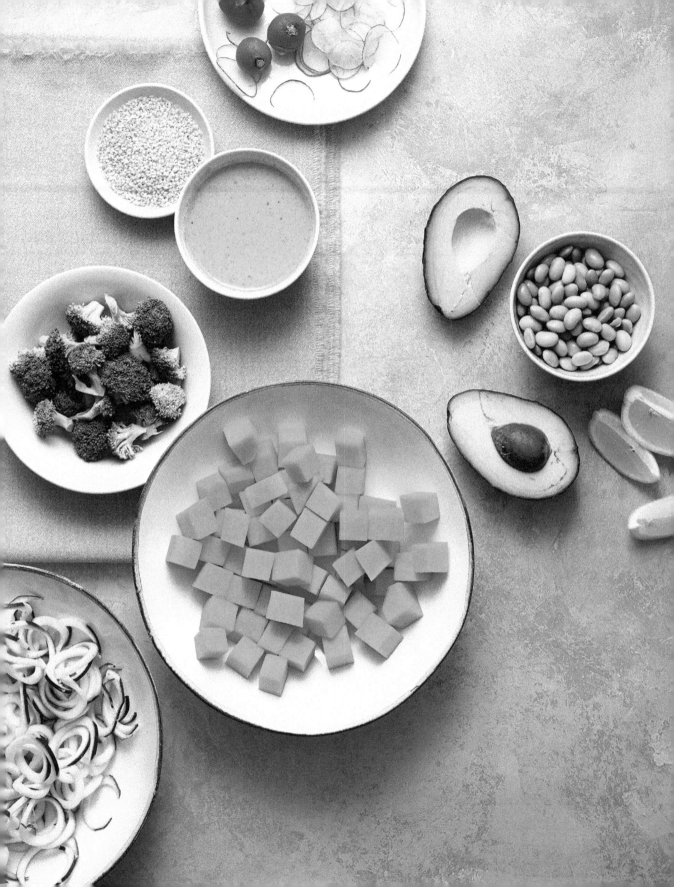

CONTENTS

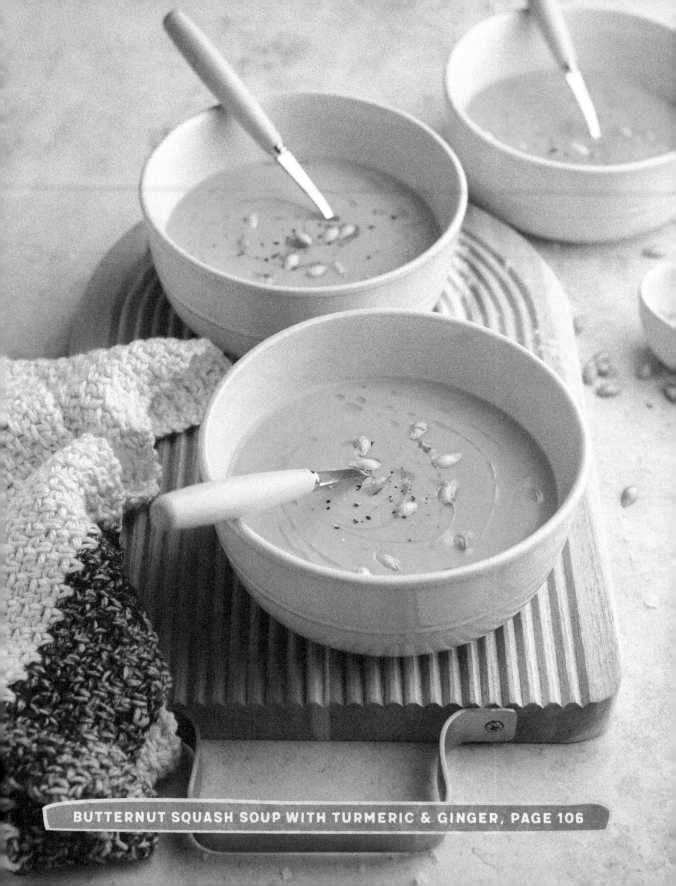

BUTTERNUT SQUASH SOUP WITH TURMERIC & GINGER, PAGE 106

INTRODUCTION

You're about to begin a clear path that will allow you to thrive on the vegan keto diet. And it's not as complicated or contradictory as you might think. If you're new to the keto diet, the idea of adding vegan into the mix might feel a little overwhelming, but rest easy, because we're here to help. Within these pages, the two of us (Whitney and Nicole) share our experience with and passion for a low-carb, plant-based diet. We're always on the hunt for foods that make us feel our best. We want to flourish, and we wish the same for you, too.

Our collective journey to this book was more than 20 years in the making.

Whitney experimented with variations of the plant-based diet for many years in an attempt to look and feel her best. She went raw vegan for a few months in 2004. In 2012, she tried out the popular high-carb, low-fat diet often referred to as 80/10/10, and in mid-2018 she dove into vegan keto. Whitney turned to the diet originally to help her lose weight. Not only did the pounds come off, but she soon experienced a decrease in inflammation and a major improvement in digestion. She found it much easier than expected to combine vegan and keto; she loved eating more fats and felt relieved when her sugar cravings diminished. This way of eating just feels right to her, in a way that few diets have felt before.

Nicole adopted a vegan keto diet after she tried to donate blood but was turned away due to a low iron count. After doing some research, she discovered that high-fat, low-grain, iron-rich foods would help boost her type O-positive blood. Nicole adopted these dietary changes over the next 10 days, then made another attempt to donate blood; this time she wasn't turned away. During her keto experiment, Nicole noticed a big increase in energy and focus. That was all the inspiration she needed to start creating delicious low-carb recipes so others could reap the same benefits.

Now that we've successfully adopted a vegan ketogenic eating plan, we want to share our knowledge with you. In this book, you'll receive practical advice on how to start and stay on the diet, including helpful meal plans, shopping lists, and 75 delicious recipes. We'll guide you through any confusion you might be feeling along the way, and we'll help you optimize the way you eat. It's our goal to help you feel and look your best every day.

By the end of this book, you'll have a greater understanding of the vegan keto diet and tools to make it work, plus tons of resources to learn more.

You've got this, so let's dive in!

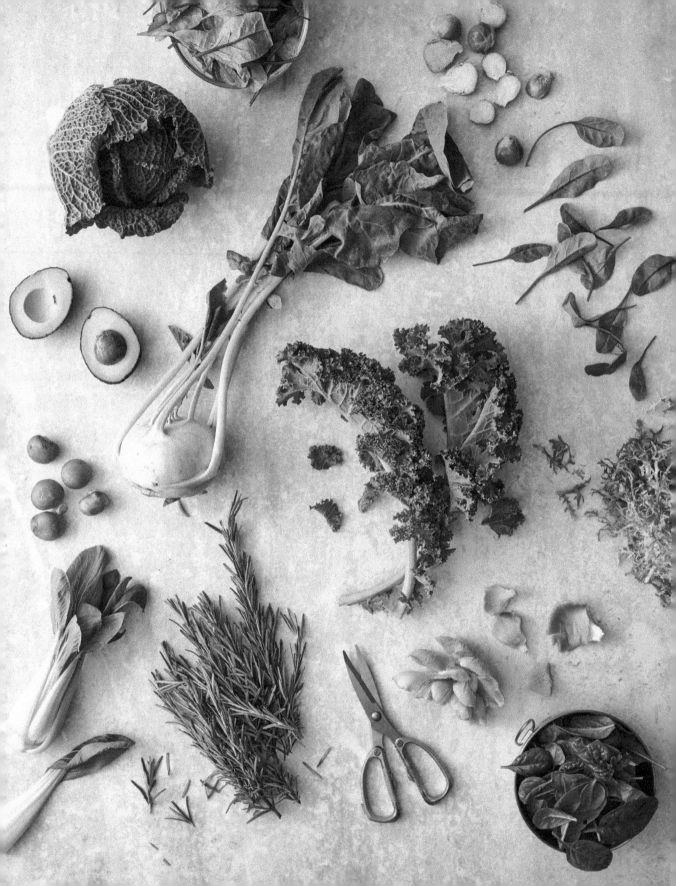

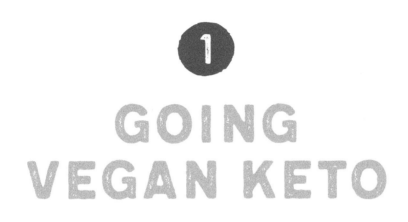

GOING VEGAN KETO

Congratulations on embarking on the vegan keto journey. Picking up this book shows a commitment to better understanding how your food choices can help you feel your best and achieve your healthiest self. In these pages, you'll find everything you need to know in order to get started right away.

A vegan keto diet focuses on low-carb vegetables, nuts, seeds, and low-glycemic fruits. As you'll see in the upcoming sections and recipes, there's plenty of variety in these food groups, so you won't have feelings of deprivation, hunger, and cravings. You can look forward to the many benefits to eating this way, including increased energy, mental clarity, sounder sleep, clearer skin, decreased inflammation, improved digestion, better hormonal function, and balanced weight.

WHY VEGAN KETO?

There's never been a better time to try the vegan keto diet. There's an ever-expanding variety of low-carb, high-fat, plant-based products on grocery store shelves. Even restaurants are embracing the trend and offering satisfying keto dishes, some of which are already vegan, and the remaining, easy to modify. Walk into the market and you'll find low net-carb food bars, zucchini noodles, cauliflower rice, unsweetened pea protein milk, and plant-based burgers bursting with protein—some of the staples of a flavorful vegan keto diet. Every week there's something new to try, so you'll never get bored with the power of plants.

Sure, on the surface, a vegan keto diet seems contradictory. A traditional ketogenic diet is often associated with an abundance of animal-based, high-fat products such as bacon, eggs, cheese, and butter. However, many vegan and keto foods cross over in a Venn diagram-like fashion. Both diets celebrate avocado, coconut, macadamia nuts, leafy greens, nuts, high-quality oils, and many other delicious ingredients. Studies have also found that each diet leads to healthy weight loss. Vegan keto unifies the best of both worlds: fiber-full, cholesterol-free, nutrient-dense plants, cruelty-free protein, and good fats—a super diet by any definition.

Eating vegan means avoiding animal products—processed or whole. Avoiding meat and dairy can have many positive benefits on your health, such as preventing or reversing heart disease and diabetes. Plus, plant-based foods are naturally free of cholesterol and packed with fiber. The vegan diet also reduces your carbon footprint, eliminates a great deal of animal suffering, and has a positive ripple effect on people around the world. Cheers to being healthier, kinder, and eco-friendlier!

The Perks of Eating Vegan Keto

- **Increased energy:** Energy is produced in the body when mitochondria break down nutrients. According to a 2006 study published in *Annals of Neurology,* and a 2008 study in *Biochimica et Biophysica Acta,* the ketogenic diet can increase the number of mitochondria, assisting cellular function and enhancing the production of fuel so the body can thrive.

- **Stabilized blood sugar:** A 2013 review of various studies on the ketogenic diet in the journal *Nutrition and Metabolism* revealed that when the body gets its energy from fat instead of glucose, blood sugar is more balanced.

- **Reduced inflammation:** According to research by immunology expert Thirumala-Devi Kanneganti and published in a 2017 article in *The New England Journal of Medicine*, ketones can help inhibit inflammatory reactions in the body.

- **Reduced cravings:** A 2014 analysis by the International Association for the Study of Obesity concluded that the ketogenic diet can help control hunger and prevent an increase in appetite. The high amounts of fat and fiber in plant-based, low-carb meals keep cravings at bay and make you feel fuller longer.

- **Weight loss and balanced weight:** In a 24-week study conducted in 2004 and published in the *Annals of Internal Medicine*, a group of overweight test subjects on a ketogenic diet lost more weight than those following a low-fat diet. Another study from 2014 published in the *International Journal of Environmental Research and Public Health* found that this way of eating can improve fat oxidative metabolism, thereby reducing body weight.

- **Reduced risk of major disease:** Clinical trials, such as a 2017 study published in *JMIR Diabetes*, found that the symptoms of type 2 diabetes can be reversed through a ketogenic diet in as little as ten weeks. Other studies, such as one from 2017, published in the *Journal of Geriatric Cardiology*, demonstrated similar benefits of plant-based diets in treating type 2 diabetes. Additionally, this diet can lower the risk of cancer, heart disease, and neurological illness, which Dr. Will Cole has written about in great detail in his book *Ketotarian*.

- **Healthier planet:** Countless data has been collected about the positive planetary impact of a plant-based diet. The United Nation's Intergovernmental Panel on Climate Change has published multiple reports urging the population to cut back on eating meat and dairy.

Many vegans overload on carbohydrates such as beans, high-sugar fruits, and grains, and refined/processed foods such as pasta, sandwiches, packaged snacks, juices, sodas, baked goods, and sugary treats. According to the US Department of Agriculture, the average person consumes over 250 grams of carbs per day. While these foods have health benefits, they can be challenging to digest, lead to spikes in blood sugar, and result in energy crashes. A diet containing excess carbohydrates can also result in insulin resistance and chronic inflammation; contributing factors for many diseases, including premature aging.

Fortunately, focusing more on healthy fats through a vegan keto diet gives your body a chance to regain its sensitivity to insulin. Dr. Joseph Mercola, an osteopathic physician, fellow of the American College of Nutrition, and author of several books, including *Fat for Fuel* and *Effortless Healing*, has concluded that foods rich in fat and protein are a more sustainable, cleaner energy source for the body than sugar from carbohydrates. Additionally, fat helps satisfy the desire for food, and consuming a high percentage of fat helps reduce cravings. If improved digestion and a balanced weight—with less abdominal fat—are your goals, the vegan keto diet could be exactly what you need to get you there.

Starting and maintaining a vegan keto diet does require intention. Change is hard, especially when it comes to switching up eating habits. But this book is going to make it easier for you, because it's loaded with tips and tricks.

WHAT IS KETO?

A ketogenic diet is a low-carbohydrate, moderate-protein, high-fat way of eating. Simply put, it can help you switch from burning sugar for fuel to burning fat for fuel. If it sounds familiar, that's because keto is not too different from the Atkins diet, the main difference being that keto requires less protein and focuses more on high-quality food.

Keto is more than a trendy diet; it's been shown to be effective against some major ailments and lifestyle challenges including obesity, high blood pressure, diabetes, cancer, and some neurological illnesses. A 2019 study published in the *Journal of Clinical Investigation Insight* found that even a modest restriction in carbs is enough to reverse heart disease, stroke, and type 2 diabetes in some people. This diet gained therapeutic renown in the 1920s when it was used by doctors to treat epilepsy.

The diet gets its name from a fat-burning metabolic state called ketosis. Molecules called ketones are produced in the liver and help with beneficial processes such as energy production, brain function, inflammation regulation, and immune system maintenance. Getting into and staying in this state requires a minimal intake of carbohydrates, which typically means consuming no more than 50 net carbs a day.

Net carbs are calculated by subtracting fiber and sugar alcohols from the total carb count of a food. For instance, if a food contains 10 grams of carbs and has 2 grams of fiber and 3 grams of erythritol, the total net carbs would be 5 grams. We will have more details about keto macronutrients in the section called All about Macronutrients (page 6).

Nutritional ketosis is not to be confused with ketoacidosis, a life-threatening condition that can develop when insulin levels are too low in a person with type 1 diabetes. Even though the keto diet is a generally safe diet that works for many people, we recommend speaking with a medical professional or healthcare provider before starting the diet to ensure it is the right fit for your body.

HOW THE VEGAN KETO DIET WORKS

Simply put, the keto diet changes how the body turns food into energy. It works like this: When fed a high-fat, low-carb, and moderate-protein diet, the body transitions into ketosis—a metabolic state that causes the liver to convert fat into fuel. By-products called ketone bodies are produced, and they help stabilize blood sugar, regulate insulin levels, and break down body fat. There are three types of ketones: acetoacetate, beta-hydroxybutyric acid, and acetone, which can be measured through blood, breath, or urine.

Keto is practically the opposite of conventional diets, in which energy is created from the sugar in carbohydrates (aka glucose). When not being used as fuel, glucose is stored as body fat. Consuming too much simple sugar can lead to insulin resistance and potentially to metabolic conditions such as diabetes and heart disease.

The vegan keto diet provides the added benefit of no cholesterol from animal products, plus a higher intake of vitamins, minerals, antioxidants, and fiber from plant-based food. As a result, the body may have lower total cholesterol and blood pressure, which can reduce the risk of many chronic diseases, including cancer.

All about Macronutrients

While many people perceive keto as a restrictive diet, it's less about specific rules and more about math. The body enters into the ketosis state when it receives a specific ratio of the three macronutrients, often referred to as macros. These are fat, protein, and carbohydrates. A typical keto diet derives 70 to 80 percent of one's daily total calories from high-quality fats, 5 to 15 percent from carbohydrates, and the remainder from protein. In contrast, the average diet comprises 20 to 35 percent fat, 46 to 65 percent carbohydrates, and 10 to 35 percent protein. Don't stress about the numbers because there are some great tools to help you with that, listed in the 7 Tips for Success section (page 22).

Fats: If you're used to a high-carb diet, it may feel challenging to get the majority of your calories from fat, but you'll quickly learn to enjoy this satisfying macronutrient. Delicious sources of fat, such as macadamia nuts, avocados, and coconut oil, will make up for the sugars you're used to consuming whenever you're hungry or have cravings.

Proteins: Getting enough protein on a vegan keto diet is easy, because you don't need much of it; just 5 to 25 percent. A variety of nuts and seeds, such as almonds, cashews, chia, hemp, and sesame seeds, are your best bet because they're low-carb. You can also enjoy moderate amounts of tofu and tempeh. Try not to rely on protein to replace the calories you would get from carbohydrates; a diet too high in protein can have some health drawbacks, such as impairing kidney function. High protein intake can also make it difficult to burn fat effectively. Many health professionals recommend getting 10 to 20 percent of your calories from protein.

Carbohydrates: When you're just starting on the diet, to get into and stay in ketosis you'll want to keep your net carbs—total carbohydrates minus fiber—within a 20- to 35-gram range. Once you've been in ketosis for a few weeks, you can up your total net carbs to 50 grams, if you prefer. Remember, there's nothing bad or wrong with fruits and high-carb vegetables. Whole foods such as sweet potatoes, brown rice, black beans, and mangos are very nutritious. However, if you want the physical benefits of a fat-burning diet, it's important to keep such foods to a minimum, at least for the first few months of keto.

As with most things in life, it's important to prioritize quality over quantity, and the same is true with your macros. In an upcoming section, you'll receive a list of essential foods to stock in your kitchen to ensure you're eating well.

Getting to Ketosis

Transitioning to ketosis can feel a little daunting at first, especially if you're used to an eating routine that places a high priority on carbs. But it's actually quite simple to achieve, when you follow the basic guidelines. If you stick to the approximate 75:20:5 ratio of fats, proteins, and carbohydrates, and keep track so you consume no more than 50 net carbs a day, you should get into ketosis quite easily. Ketosis can also be achieved through fasting, but a low-carb diet is a gentler route. The time it takes to enter into ketosis depends on your body and dietary choices, but on average it will take several days to a few weeks.

It's also important to know that the ideal macro ratio depends on the individual. Factors such as age, weight, activity level, and dietary history impact how your body responds to food. That's why it's important not to be too rigid with the numbers. Instead, focus on results. We've compiled recipes and meal plans to help you get into ketosis with ease.

The best way to know when you've entered ketosis is to test your breath, urine, or blood. You can do this through various methods, such as pH strips, breath devices that measure acetone, and blood meters (more on this in the next section). You may notice physical signs that tell you you're in ketosis, such as mental clarity, increased energy, clearer skin, more restful sleep, decreased bloating, and fewer cravings, but to be sure, it's best to test.

If you're struggling to get into ketosis, there are a couple of "shortcuts" you can take. Start by limiting net carbs to 20 to 35 grams a day, especially if you've been eating upward of 50 grams. It's also helpful to consume MCT oil, usually derived from coconut. (MCT stands for medium-chain triglycerides.) This concentrated super fuel goes directly to the liver to be used for energy production.

Staying in Ketosis

Once you're committed to vegan keto, you'll find it fairly easy to stay in ketosis. After tracking your meals for a few weeks, you'll acquire an intuition for macros and where your body's at throughout each day. However, if you want to ensure that you're in the ketosis state, it's best to test yourself with one of the following methods.

Urine test: You can measure your levels by urinating on ketone strips, which will display a color to indicate whether you're in ketosis or not. This is an affordable method that offers quick results, but it's not the most reliable.

Breath test: You can purchase a device that measures acetone, a by-product of ketones, in your breath. This device can be pricy and isn't perfectly accurate.

Blood test: This method involves using a device to prick your finger to quickly get a ketone reading. The device and test strips are quite expensive and it's slightly uncomfortable to use; however, it is the most accurate way to test.

Factors other than your diet can affect your ability to stay in ketosis. Intermittent fasting can be beneficial to the process, which typically means eating within an 8-hour window and fasting for 16 hours. Please consult your doctor if you plan to start intermittent fasting while on a ketogenic diet. It's also important to keep stress at a minimum and get plenty of sleep each night, as stress and lack of sleep can sabotage your willpower and throw off your eating habits.

Keep in mind that it's not ideal for most people to be on a continuous keto diet. Several well-known medical professionals—such as clinic doctor Mark Hyman, board-certified family physician Joseph Mercola, and functional medicine provider Anthony Gustin—recommend getting into ketosis intermittently (for two to eight weeks) and then cycling in higher amounts of carbohydrates and proteins, plus doing periods of partial fasting. If you continue keto indefinitely, the benefits could decrease and may even be reversed.

The optimal goal with keto is to achieve metabolic flexibility so you can burn fat as fuel. After your first month or two in ketosis, you can have occasional higher net-carb days, eating between 100 to 150 grams. This means you can enjoy starchy foods such as sweet potatoes, rice, and quinoa again. On these days, you should balance out your macro ratios, being mindful to reduce your fat intake based on the amount of carbohydrates and protein you add. You can do this two to three times a week, ideally after vigorous exercise.

"KETO FLU"—SIGNS AND SYMPTOMS

Often in the first few weeks of a ketogenic diet, some people experience something called the "keto flu." You may experience this as a lack of energy, brain fog, headaches, intense hunger, nausea, trouble sleeping, upset stomach, and/or irritable mood. Other side effects include constipation (usually due to increased fats), decreased libido, and decreased physical performance. What's happening is this: You're basically going through a short-term detox period during which your body switches from burning sugar for fuel to fat. It's a significant physical adjustment to decrease carbohydrates, and your metabolism is going through a big shift. Your fat cells may release stored heavy metals and chemicals, and your gut bacteria will change.

We know, these symptoms don't make keto very appealing. The good news is, not everyone goes through this and it doesn't last too long for those who do. The even better news is that there are ways to prevent or relieve the symptoms.

Staying thoroughly hydrated is very important. Regular physical exercise such as walking, running, and yoga will keep your organs and muscles in great shape. Make sure you get plenty of rest, too, so your body can repair itself while you sleep. It's also helpful to ensure you're getting enough mineral-rich salt in your diet, and consuming foods rich in electrolytes, especially before and after moving your body. Lastly, if you're not feeling ideal, you might need to increase your fat intake. Consuming coconut oil is a great shortcut for doing so.

Even if you don't have any tough physical symptoms, you might experience some strong emotions, ranging from euphoria to frustration and/or feeling overwhelmed. Stay patient and positive during this big transition. Keep a food diary and/or journal to track what you're going through, and know that this, too, shall pass.

COMMON CONCERNS

Embarking on a vegan keto diet requires determination, planning, and detachment from previous eating habits. Don't let this transition discourage you. Instead, let it empower you. With the right mindset and commitment, the benefits of a vegan keto diet far outweigh any temporary challenges. If you're feeling hesitant or fearful due to some preconceived notions about this way of eating, this section is designed to put your mind at ease. You've got this.

"It's just a fad diet that's not sustainable." Many people are drawn to the keto diet because they've heard that it's an effective way to lose weight. Once they give it a try and achieve the physical results they want, some people revert back to their old ways of eating and gain the weight back. However, you can sustain the health benefits. Instead of viewing vegan keto as a quick fix through a few weeks of deprivation, think of it as an enjoyable lifestyle choice. Talk to a healthcare provider to help you determine how long you should stay on the diet, and read up on the benefits of carbohydrate-loading, as mentioned in the following pages.

"I can't live without fruit!" The keto diet generally does not include fruit because of its high sugar content, so if you're a big fan of nature's candy, this may be challenging. The good news is that berries are an option, so you can still get your fix. Citrus fruits are another possibility; try lemons, limes, and grapefruits. Plus, once you've been in ketosis for a month or two and have become fat-adapted, you could try carbohydrate-loading. Also known as "refeeding" within the keto community, this is when you pick a day or two during the week to enjoy higher-carb foods such as fruits. If you have an insatiable craving outside these days, opt for small servings of lower-fructose fruits such as cantaloupe, honeydew melon, kiwi, passion fruit, or pineapple. Keto is more about the macronutrient ratio than it is about "right" and "wrong" foods, so don't feel that you must be dogmatic about what you eat.

"The diet is so restrictive; I'll get bored." When you switch to a diet that feels more restrictive than your usual diet, you may find yourself craving higher-carb foods for a bit. However, transitioning to any diet gets easier over time, and "off-limit" foods become less tempting. You'll become more creative with your food choices and learn to enjoy them more than ever. Simply switching up an ingredient or two or adding something extra into a recipe can make it taste completely different. Try different varieties of foods; for instance, there are several types of avocado, each with a unique taste and texture. Get adventurous with your shopping lists and recipes and experiment with your meal plan. Take the occasional break from cooking to treat yourself to vegan keto meals at restaurants and packaged foods from grocery stores.

"I won't be able to dine out." Fortunately, many establishments now offer low-carb dishes. You can find some at most Thai restaurants, such as coconut soups and red or green curry (without rice). If you're dining with a group and they pick a place that isn't vegan keto-friendly, most restaurants can make modifications to get you close to a vegan keto dish. Salads are a perfect example. Those with roasted low-carb veggies, nuts, seeds, and/or avocado are best, and make sure they're dressed with a generous amount of olive oil.

"But fat is bad!" In a 2004 study from the *Annals of Internal Medicine*, researchers concluded that the body runs more efficiently on fats than sugars. It's important to speak with your doctor and get some bloodwork done to determine if a higher fat diet is a safe choice for your body. If you get medical approval to try keto, track how you feel and look after a few months, and use those results to reflect on your previous opinion about fat. Also, remember that not all fat is created equally. The dishes in this book are centered around high-quality ingredients with an abundance of health benefits.

DON'T FORGET ABOUT YOUR MICRONUTRIENTS

As with any diet, it's important to be mindful of vitamins and minerals to ensure optimal physical function. Fortunately, you'll easily acquire most micronutrients through eating plants. Variety is the key here, so be sure to stock up on as many of these powerful foods as you can handle. Here are some important micronutrients and sources for obtaining them:

Calcium: almonds, broccoli, dark leafy greens, sesame seeds, and tofu

Iodine: sea vegetables and iodized salt

Iron: cashews, leafy greens, sesame seeds, sunflower seeds, pumpkin seeds, tempeh, and tofu

Magnesium: dark chocolate, pine nuts, potassium-rich greens, and seeds (hemp, chia, pumpkin)

Omega-3 fatty acids: chia seeds, flax seeds, olive oil, spirulina, and walnuts

Potassium: almonds, artichokes, avocados, broccoli, hemp seeds, mushrooms, spinach, and Swiss chard

Vitamin A: broccoli and leafy greens such as spinach and kale

Vitamin D: mushrooms, plant-based milk, and tofu

Vitamin K2: fermented foods

Vitamin B12: fortified foods such as nutritional yeast

Zinc: chocolate (unsweetened), mushrooms, seeds (sesame, pumpkin, and flax), and spinach

Other excellent sources of micronutrients include:

Fresh or dried herbs and spices: Apart from providing great flavor, herbs and spices are rich in antioxidants and contain powerful essential oils. Enjoy basil, cilantro, chives, cinnamon, dill, ginger, mint, oregano, parsley, rosemary, thyme, and beyond.

Sprouts: Sprouted seeds, such as broccoli and alfalfa, not only add a nice crunchy texture to dishes but are also packed with nutrients.

Probiotic-rich foods: Kimchi and sauerkraut aid digestion and enhance the effects of this high-fiber diet. Fiber is a vital carbohydrate that converts to fat and can even reduce the absorption of carbohydrates. It benefits the immune system and digestion and can lower cholesterol, blood pressure, and inflammation. Aim to consume no less than 35 grams of fiber a day, with a loftier goal of 50 to 75 grams to get maximum benefit.

In general, whole foods provide a powerful nutrient punch. However, you may need some extra assistance from supplements to acquire certain vitamins, such as B12 and D (you can absorb vitamin D from the sun, but it can be difficult to get enough sunshine). Taurine, carnosine, and creatine are also challenging to get on a plant-based diet, so consider taking those supplements as well.

The amount of each nutrient you need depends on your age, gender, body size, and activity level. It's helpful to get your levels checked by a medical professional to ensure you're obtaining adequate amounts.

THE VEGAN KETO KITCHEN

Food is one of life's greatest pleasures, and you don't have to feel restricted on the vegan keto diet. A kitchen stocked with the following essentials will make preparing meals easier and more exciting. Focus on fresh, whole, unprocessed ingredients without chemical additives, and ideally choose those that are locally grown, organic, and/or non-GMO. When purchasing packaged foods, read the labels and look for items that contain no added sugar or processed ingredients, such as artificial sweeteners.

Pantry Essentials

Cocoa and cacao: Cocoa, and its raw counterpart cacao, is a fantastic source of antioxidants, magnesium, monounsaturated fat, and polyphenols. Our recipes call for cacao powder, nibs, and butter. We also recommend keeping unsweetened dark chocolate on hand for snacking and melting into some sweet treats. We've specified the different forms of chocolate needed in each recipe.

Coconut milk and coconut cream: The full-fat options show up in several of our recipes, especially drinks and desserts.

Low-carb flours: Low-carb flours will be used to make many baked goods, so make sure you have almond flour and coconut flour. These flours are high in fiber and protein, and have great consistency when used in baking. Psyllium husk, or ground seeds, such as chia and flax, are also used in some vegan keto recipes.

Nuts and nut butters: Our favorites are almonds, Brazil nuts, cashews, macadamia nuts, pecans, and walnuts. Pili nuts are a popular keto snack, so give them a try for something new and interesting.

Oils: Have a variety on hand for cooking, dressings, and sauces. Most oils are great sources of monounsaturated fat, and several contain polyphenols, which are beneficial for your gut microbiome. Stock up on coconut oil and avocado oil for sautéing and roasting, extra-virgin olive oil and sesame oil for chilled dishes, and MCT oil for boosting ketones and reducing cravings.

Seeds and seed butters: You'll use chia seeds, flax seeds, hemp seeds, psyllium seed husks, pumpkin seeds, sesame seeds and tahini, and sunflower seeds in many of our recipes.

Dried spices and other seasonings: Basil, cayenne, coconut shreds, cumin, curry powder, dill, ginger, mint, paprika, pepper, sea salt, tamari, veggie broth, turmeric, and vanilla are used generously throughout the cookbook.

Sugar-free sweeteners: These are vital for sweet treats and for enhancing the flavor of beverages. Load up on stevia powder, monk fruit crystals, and/or erythritol granules.

Vinegars: We're big fans of apple cider and rice vinegar for adding depth and balance to recipes.

Refrigerated Essentials

Fermented foods: Kimchi, pickles, and sauerkraut are good staples loaded with micronutrients beneficial to your digestive system. Tempeh, miso paste, and natto are also tasty, but should be enjoyed in moderation.

Fresh herbs: Varieties you'll use most often include basil, cilantro, dill, ginger root, lemongrass, mint, parsley, rosemary, tarragon, and thyme.

Low-carb produce: Broccoli, cauliflower, celery, cucumber, jicama, leafy greens—such as arugula, kale, salad greens, and spinach—leeks, onions, peas, peppers, mushrooms, shallots, and zucchini.

Low-glycemic fruits: Blackberries, blueberries, raspberries, and strawberries are delicious snacks and liven up many sweet recipes.

Plant-based milks: We are fans of milks made from peas, almonds, coconut, or hemp seeds for smoothies, coffee, and tea. Plus, they're used in some recipes. You can usually swap one for the other, so choose an unsweetened varietal of preference.

Nut-based cheeses: Nut-based cheeses such as those made from cashews, almonds, or macadamia nuts make a nice snack, in moderation. Be mindful of the portion size and total net carbs.

Sauces and dressings: These take vegetables to the next level. Sugar-free barbecue sauce, hot sauce, low-sugar ketchup, mustard, sugar-free salad dressings, and vegan mayonnaise are great to have on hand for quick flavor boosts.

Shirataki noodles: These are an excellent pasta alternative. Some varieties are made from tofu, but most are derived from the konjac yam. There are both refrigerated and shelf-stable versions of these noodles, and it doesn't really matter which you choose to buy.

Sprouts: Our top choice for flavor and nutrient density is broccoli sprouts, followed by mung bean, alfalfa, clover, and radish. Just be sure to purchase sprouts only when needed because they don't stay fresh very long.

Tofu, organic, firm: Tofu is made from soybeans and is fairly low in carbs, so eating it in moderation is fine.

Other Perishable Essentials

Avocado: The vegan keto dieter's best friend. In addition to being delicious on its own and in almost every recipe, it's full of high-quality fat, essential nutrients, and antioxidants that boost brain power and gut health.

Garlic: It's used in many recipes as a flavor enhancer, so make sure to stock it at all times. Fortunately, it stays fresh for quite a while.

Lemon: A versatile citrus fruit that adds acidic flavor to countless dishes, along with nutrients such as vitamin C.

Lime: Another citrus fruit that brings beverages and foods such as guacamole to life. It has a host of health benefits, especially for the skin and digestion.

Nutritional yeast: A crowd pleaser and for good reason: It tastes like cheese! Look for formulations fortified with vitamins such as B12 to get the most bang for your buck.

Onions: A kitchen staple. Have at least one on hand of each color—white, red, and yellow—as they each taste slightly different.

Seed crackers: Particularly those made from flax, are excellent crunchy snacks and can stand in for toast. Check the ingredients to ensure the brand you select doesn't contain grains such as rice. Opt for crackers that contain a variety of seeds such as chia and pumpkin.

Tea and coffee: Keto staples because they offer a boost of energy and antioxidants and can suppress the appetite without adding calories. If you prefer tea, we recommend matcha green tea powder because it packs a one-two punch of flavor and nutrition.

Tomatoes: Great color, plus they add important vitamins, minerals, and antioxidants to your meals. Check the recipes in case they call for specific varieties such as vine, Roma, or cherry; each have a slightly different flavor and texture. Enjoy in moderation.

Vegan protein powder: Made from protein sources such as pea, hemp, and/or pumpkin seed, these powders can be used in baked goods and smoothies, and on their own mixed with water as a protein-packed meal replacement.

FOOD TO ENJOY VS. FOODS TO AVOID

	ENJOY	IN MODERATION	AVOID
VEGETABLES	leafy greens (e.g., spinach, kale, chard, lettuces, arugula); cruciferous vegetables (e.g., broccoli, cauliflower, Brussels sprouts); bell peppers, celery, mushrooms, asparagus, artichokes, cabbage, cucumber, zucchini, bok choy, radishes, kohlrabi, sprouts (alfalfa, broccoli), sea vegetables (wakame, dulse, nori, kelp, spirulina)	carrots, pumpkin and other winter squashes, onions, garlic, okra, snap peas, green beans, nightshades (eggplant, tomatoes)	potatoes, sweet potatoes, yams, corn, parsnips, plantains, taro
SEEDS & NUTS	chia seeds, flax seeds, hemp seeds, pumpkin seeds, sesame seeds, psyllium seeds, sunflower seeds; pecans, Brazil nuts, almonds, macadamia nuts, hazelnuts, walnuts	cashews, pine nuts peanuts, pistachios	quinoa, millet
FATS & OILS	avocado oil, coconut oil, extra virgin olive oil, MCT oil, cocoa/cacao butter	canola oil, vegetable oil, peanut oil, soybean oil	all animal fats, including butter and cheese; corn oil, cottonseed oil, safflower oil
FRUITS	avocados, olives, coconut, citrus fruits (lemon, lime)	berries, grapefruit, jackfruit	all other fruits (e.g., bananas, apples, pineapples, grapes, etc.), dried fruits

	ENJOY	IN MODERATION	AVOID
GRAINS & FLOURS	coconut, nut flours		wheat, rice, corn, oats, rye, spelt, barley, buckwheat, amaranth, cereal, arrowroot, cassava flour
ANIMAL PRODUCTS: MEAT & SEAFOOD	none	none	all (no meat, fish, dairy, eggs, gelatin, etc.)
SWEETENERS, SPICES & SEASONINGS	stevia, monk fruit, sugar alcohols (sorbitol, erythritol, xylitol), nutritional yeast, fresh and dried herbs (basil, rosemary, etc.), spices (e.g., cinnamon), mustard, hot sauce, apple cider vinegar	artificial sweeteners (e.g., sucralose-based), sugar-free BBQ sauce	added sugar, agave nectar, brown rice syrup, maple syrup, honey, molasses, date sugar, coconut sugar or nectar, corn syrup, malt, balsamic vinegar
BEVERAGES	water, tea, coffee, sparkling water, unsweetened milks made from nuts, seeds, or peas, keto smoothies (see recipes)	dry red wine, vodka, unsweetened milks made from legumes (e.g., soy)	other alcohols, soda, kombucha
LEGUMES / BEANS	None	edamame, tempeh, tofu, natto, miso, peas, tamari	hummus, lentils, chickpeas, kidney beans, black beans, pinto beans, white beans, soybeans, etc.

EQUIPMENT AND TOOLS

Before we dive into the meal plans and recipes, let's take a look at what you might need in terms of kitchen equipment and tools.

Must-Haves

Baking sheets: A trio of baking sheets is a good starting point, in either stainless steel or silicone.

Cutting board: Large in size and ideally made from wood

High-powered blender: A high-speed machine that works efficiently and effectively

Knives: A ceramic chef's knife, a small paring knife, and a serrated knife for slicing tomatoes

Measuring cups and spoons: A set of each for precise measuring of ingredients

Mixing bowls: Glass or silicone, in a variety of sizes

Pots and pans: A 2- to 3-quart pot and a 10- to 12-inch skillet or saucepan. Stainless steel, ceramic, or cast iron is ideal. Nonstick pans can release chemicals during cooking and cleaning, so it's best to avoid those unless they are free of PFOA, PTFE, and cadmium.

Spatula and spoons: A variety of sizes in both wood and silicone

Spiralizer: If you enjoy veggie noodles, such as those made from zucchini, this tool will save you money in the long run.

Storage containers: For leftovers, meal prep, and storing food. Stainless steel, glass, ceramic, or BPA-free plastic are best.

Strainer: Needed for rinsing ingredients and straining low-carb noodles

Nice-to-Haves

Baking dish: An 8-inch pan for baked goods or roasting vegetables

Garlic peeler: A time saver that also reduces the smell of garlic on your fingers

Grater and/or zester: For grating vegetables or zesting citrus

Immersion blender: Sometimes referred to as a hand blender, it's useful for pureeing soups in pots.

Lemon juicer: Perfect for getting every last drop of the lemon juice quickly without worrying about the seeds

Mandoline slicer: For uniformly sliced veggies

Muffin tin: To make keto treats that need to hold their shape; also great for portion control

Nut milk bag: A soft strainer made from mesh material, used for making plant-based milks, such as almond or cashew

Pickling jars with sealing lids: Perfect for pickling and fermenting foods but can also be used as airtight, glass storage containers

Silicone baking mat: An eco-friendly alternative to parchment paper that helps prevent foods sticking to baking sheets

7 TIPS FOR SUCCESS

As with any lifestyle change, there will be some challenges as you embark on the vegan keto diet. But don't let them discourage you; there are ways to meet those challenges. Here are our top seven tips to succeed:

1. **Remember your intention.** The best ways to maintain a commitment is to remember why you're doing it and acknowledge your progress. Write down your reasons for starting this diet; if you have moments of weakness or frustration you can look back at this statement, which will help you tap into your willpower to stay committed. Don't stress. You don't have to do keto perfectly. If you fall off the wagon, just get right back on as soon as you can.

2. **Begin every week by looking at your schedule.** Use the meal plans in the next chapter to help you decide what to eat and when, then do some meal prep in advance if that feels beneficial. Stock up on snacks that you can grab in hangry moments. If you have plans to dine out, determine which low-carb, plant-based dishes are on the restaurant menu (see Common Concerns, page 10).

3. **Track your food intake.** There are many mobile apps and website calculators that can help you do the math to fine-tune your ratios. Input each meal you eat into them to learn the macronutrient and micronutrient details. Our top recommendations are MyFitnessPal, Cronometer, Lifesum, Carb Manager, and The Keto Diet App. In addition to helping you calculate nutrients, several of these types of tools will also give you dietary tips based on your physical stats and goals.

4. **Embrace Internet food shopping.** By planning ahead and ordering items online, you can save money and keep your kitchen stocked with exactly what you need. Our go-to brands are listed in the Resources section on page 151.

5. **Have a craving for something sweet or experiencing hunger pangs?** Try a Cookie Fat Bomb (page 82). You can also eat a tablespoon of coconut oil or MCT oil to reduce hunger and boost energy (or mix it into coffee or tea if you're not keen on downing a spoonful). Coffee is

a great appetite suppressor and can be a tasty treat when mixed with a sugar substitute (such as monk fruit) and unsweetened milk. Chia seeds can also tide you over; mix them into beverages or make a simple chia pudding.

6. **Make keto fun!** This diet is growing in popularity and there's a big benefit to that: new food products to tantalize your taste buds. Make an adventure out of hunting for items at the grocery store (or online). Keto goodies are sprinkled throughout most markets. Check packages for "low carb," "grain free," and "paleo," the latter of which are sometimes keto, too. Read ingredient lists to ensure that products don't contain anything you should be avoiding. (See Foods to Enjoy vs. Foods to Avoid on page 18 for more guidance.)

7. **Focus on how you feel instead of how you look.** If you are trying out vegan keto to lose weight, we wish you the best of luck with reaching your goal. However, as you've learned, there are so many other physical benefits to this way of eating beyond your appearance. How you feel on the inside is ultimately more important than how you look on the outside, so consider weight loss a bonus rather than the most important factor.

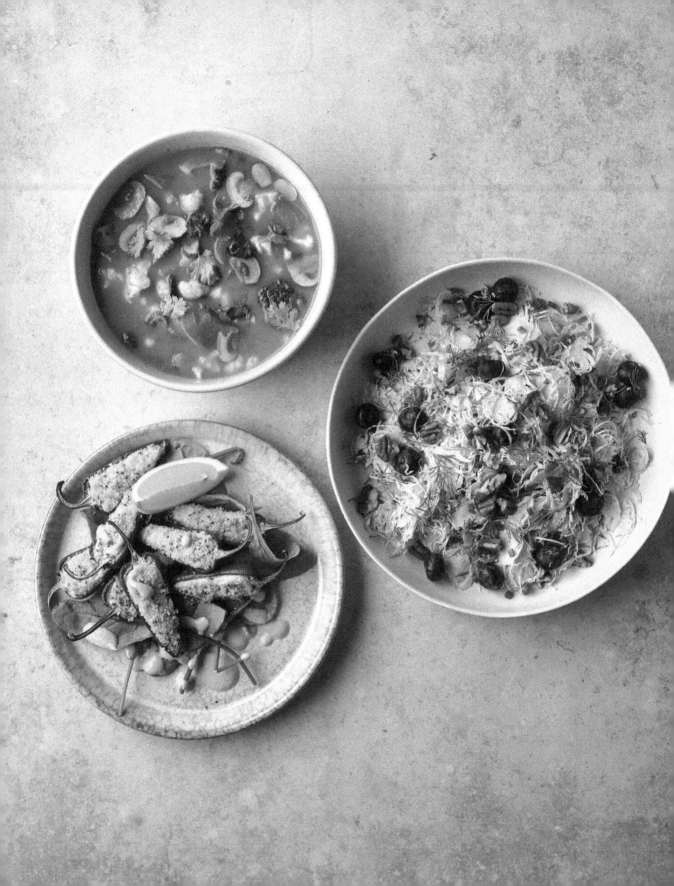

VEGAN KETO MEAL PLANS

Meal planning is a fantastic way to save time, money—and frustration. We want vegan keto to be as easy as possible for you, so we compiled two weeks of daily food suggestions—including breakfast, lunch, and dinner—based on the recipes in this book. We also provide a shopping list and snack ideas to eliminate confusion and keep hunger at bay. All you have to do is buy the ingredients for the week and follow the plan. Having everything laid out will really help keep you on track, especially if you're new to this way of eating, and by the end of the plan, you should be in ketosis.

Ideally, choose one day to look at the week ahead—our plan is based on that day being Sunday, but choose whichever day works best for you. Plan your grocery shopping, and perhaps make some dishes in advance so you can grab them whenever it's mealtime. An asterisk (*) next to a dish means you can make it ahead of time. Some days include leftovers from the previous day to give you a break from the kitchen; those meals are noted in *italics*. Depending on your flavor preferences, appetite, and schedule, your meal planning may look slightly different from ours, and that's fine. We encourage you to experiment so you can discover the food types and amounts that fit into your life. Feel free to swap out a dish or two to your liking.

This list has been designed to be simple and budget-friendly. These items will be used in the upcoming recipes, so all you need to do is purchase them and you'll be ready for food prep. If some items seem pricey, keep in mind that these are upfront costs for ingredients you'll use over and over to make nutritious and delicious food.

SNACK IDEAS

Before we get to the specific meal plans, we want to provide an abundance of snack ideas for both weeks. Choose one or two snacks a day to tide you over between meals. These are especially useful if you're exercising frequently and need additional calories.

EASY SNACKS YOU CAN MAKE

(brands we like are in parentheses)

- Avocado on flaxseed crackers (Foods Alive and Doctor in the Kitchen)
- Berries mixed into unsweetened coconut yogurt (GT's Living Foods Cocoyo)
- Guacamole and raw veggies
- Sliced cucumber with tahini, salt, and nutritional yeast

SNACK RECIPES FROM THIS BOOK

- Cookie Fat Bombs (page 82)
- Zucchini Chips (page 70)
- Gourmet "Cheese" Balls (page 74)
- Avocado "Fries" (page 76)
- Fresh Rosemary Keto Bread (page 80) with avocado
- Smoky "Hummus" and Veggies (page 78)
- Turmeric Cauliflower "Pickles" (page 71)
- Raw Keto Ranch (page 43) with broccoli florets and celery

PACKAGED SNACKS (brands we like are in parentheses)

- Lupini beans (BRAMI)
- Bars made with vegan keto ingredients (Bhu Foods, Dang, No Cow, and Love Good Fats)
- Dehydrated snacks such as kale chips and broccoli bites (Rhythm Superfoods)
- Refrigerated vegan keto drinks (Cave Shake, Kiito, or Koia)
- Low-sugar, vegan candy (Jealous Sweets, Smart Sweets gelatin-free treats, or Eating Evolved keto cups)
- Protein chips (Protes)
- Seaweed snacks (Sea Snacks nori sheets)

SINGLE-INGREDIENT SNACKS

- Berries (blueberries, strawberries, raspberries, blackberries)
- Nuts (almonds, macadamia nuts)
- Olives
- Pickles
- Seeds

WEEK 1 MEAL PLAN

	NET CARBS · FAT · PROTEIN	BREAKFAST
MONDAY	43g · 114g · 63g	Market Veggie Tofu Scramble (page 66)
TUESDAY	40g · 84g · 22g	Go Get 'Em Green Smoothie Bowl (page 57)
WEDNESDAY	43g · 140g · 37g	Avocado Boats with Flax Crackers (page 62)
THURSDAY	40g · 69g · 34g	*Market Veggie Tofu Scramble*
FRIDAY	37g · 106g · 33g	Go Get 'Em Green Smoothie Bowl
SATURDAY	35g · 103g · 35g	*Chia Parfait (page 55)
SUNDAY	32g · 89g · 24g	Almond and Vanilla Pancakes (page 60)

LUNCH	SNACK	DINNER
Keto Cobb Salad (page 96)	*Cookie Fat Bombs (page 82)	Cauliflower-Stuffed Green Peppers (page 134)
Kale, Avocado & Tahini Salad (page 94) *Tomato Bisque (page 103)	*Zucchini Chips (page 70)	Smoked Shiitake Thai Lettuce Cups (page 120)
Citrus Arugula Salad (page 90) *Tuscan Kale Soup (page 110)	*Cookie Fat Bombs	Shirataki Noodles Carbonara (page 132)
Raw Tabouli (page 86) Italian Wedding Soup (page 111)	Smoky "Hummus" and Veggies (page 78)	Rainbow Kebabs (page 136)
Kale, Avocado & Tahini Salad Tomato Bisque	*Turmeric Cauliflower "Pickles" (page 71)	Cauliflower-Stuffed Green Peppers
Vegan Niçoise Salad (page 95) Gazpacho (page 102)	*Cookie Fat Bombs	Shirataki Noodles Carbonara
Ranch Wedge Salad with Coconut "Bacon" (page 98)	*Turmeric Cauliflower "Pickles"	Keto Margherit-o Pizza (page 126)

WEEK 1 SHOPPING LIST

FATS & OILS

- Almond butter (4¼ cups)
- Cashews, raw (1 cup)
- Chia seeds (⅜ cup)
- Coconut flakes, unsweet-ened (4 cups)
- Coconut oil (1 cup)
- Flaxseed, ground (2 tablespoons)
- Hemp seeds (1¾ cups)
- MCT oil (3 tablespoons)
- Cold-pressed olive oil (6⅓ cups)
- Pepitas (⅜ cup)
- Pine nuts, dried (½ cup)
- Sesame oil (2 tablespoons)
- Walnuts, raw (4 cups)

PRODUCE

- Arugula (1 [5-ounce]) bag
- Avocados (5 medium)
- Basil, fresh (2 bunches)
- Green beans (1 pound)
- Broccoli, florets (1 pound)
- Butter leaf lettuce (2 heads)
- Butternut squash (1 whole)
- Cabbage, purple (1 head)
- Carrots (1 pound)
- Cauliflower (2 large heads)
- Cauliflower rice (4 cups)
- Celery (1 bunch)
- Chives (1 bunch)
- Cilantro, fresh (1 bunch)
- Cucumbers (2)
- Daikon radish (1)
- Garlic (4 heads)
- Ginger root, fresh (1 large piece)
- Grapefruit (½ medium)
- Green peas, frozen (2 cups)

- Mixed salad greens (8 cups)
- Jalapeño pepper (1)
- Kale (3 bunches)
- Leeks (2)
- Lemongrass (3 sticks)
- Lemons (12)
- Lettuce (1 head)
- Lettuce, romaine (1 head)
- Mint (1 bunch)
- Mushrooms (3 [8-ounce]) boxes
- Onions, yellow (2)
- Onions, red (3)
- Parsley, fresh (3 bunches)
- Bell peppers, green (5)

- Bell peppers, red (2)
- Bell peppers, yellow (1)
- Radishes (5)
- Raspberries (1 [8-ounce]) container
- Rutabaga (1)
- Scallions (1 bunch)
- Shallots (2)
- Spinach (6 pounds)
- Thyme, fresh (1 bunch)
- Tomatoes, cherry (3 [10-ounce]) containers
- Tomatoes, heirloom (4 pounds)
- Tomatoes, Roma (6)
- Zucchini (2 large)

PANTRY ITEMS (brands we like are in parentheses)

- Almond flour
- Capers
- Coconut cream
- Coconut flour
- Coconut milk, full-fat
- Cold-brew coffee (Bulletproof, Chameleon, or Four Sigmatic)

- Liquid aminos
- Liquid smoke, hickory
- Liquid stevia (Omica, Sweetleaf, or NuNaturals)
- Maple-flavored syrup (Lakanto or NuNaturals)
- Marsala wine, dry

- Miso paste
- Monk fruit sweetener (Lakanto or You Are Loved Foods)
- Mushroom broth
- Olives, black, sliced
- Psyllium husks
- Shirataki noodles (Miracle Noodles)
- Soybeans, black
- Stewed tomatoes
- Tahini
- Tamari
- Tomato paste
- Tomato sauce
- Veggie broth
- Vinegar, apple cider
- Vinegar, white
- Wakame, dried
- Wine, white

DAIRY ALTERNATIVES (brands we like are in parentheses)

- Vegan butter (2 cups) (Miyoko's or Earth Balance)
- Vegan mozzarella (24 ounces) (Miyoko's)
- Almond milk, unsweetened (7½ cups)
- Hemp milk, unsweetened (4 cups)

PROTEINS

- Tofu, firm and sprouted (4 [14-ounce] blocks)

DRIED HERBS, SPICES, AND BAKING INGREDIENTS

Tip: To save money, try to buy only the amounts you need in the bulk food section of the market. If that's not an option, purchase smaller containers whenever possible so nothing goes to waste.

- Baking powder
- Bay leaves (5)
- Basil, dried
- Black peppercorns
- Cacao powder
- Cardamom, ground
- Cayenne pepper
- Red pepper flakes
- Cinnamon, ground
- Coriander seeds
- Cumin, ground
- Cumin seeds
- Dill, dried
- Fennel seeds
- Garlic powder
- Mint, dried
- Nutmeg, ground
- Nutritional yeast
- Old Bay seasoning
- Oregano, dried
- Paprika
- Sea salt
- Sesame seeds, black
- Sun-dried tomatoes
- Turmeric powder
- Vanilla extract

WEEK 2 MEAL PLAN

	NET CARBS · FAT · PROTEIN	BREAKFAST
MONDAY	27g · 53g · 15g	*Chia Parfait (page 55)
TUESDAY	30g · 107g · 31g	Coffee Smoothie (page 54)
WEDNESDAY	43g · 137g · 38g	Avocado Boats with Flax Crackers (page 62)
THURSDAY	35g · 126g · 39g	Go Get 'Em Green Smoothie Bowl (page 57)
FRIDAY	36g · 76g · 24g	*Chia Parfait*
SATURDAY	29g · 79g · 17g	Coffee Smoothie
SUNDAY	24g · 57g · 28g	Tuscan "Quiche" Bites (page 64)

LUNCH	SNACK	DINNER
Broccoli & Raspberry "Bacon" Salad (page 89) *Creamy Leek Soup (page 105)	*Smoky "Hummus" and Veggies (page 78)	Keto Margherit-o Pizza (page 126)
Warming Spiced Chili (page 133)	Avocado "Fries" (page 76)	Big Greek Spinach Salad (page 92) *Creamy Leek Soup*
Ranch Wedge Salad with Coconut "Bacon" (page 98)	*Smoky "Hummus" and Veggies*	Good Shepherd's Pie (page 129)
Big Greek Spinach Salad	*Cookie Fat Bombs (page 82)	Cauliflower-Stuffed Green Peppers (page 134)
Citrus Arugula Salad (page 90) *Butternut Squash Soup with Turmeric & Ginger (106)	*Smoky "Hummus" and Veggies*	Rainbow Kebabs (page 136)
Ranch Wedge Salad with Coconut "Bacon" Tomato Bisque (page 103)	*Turmeric Cauliflower "Pickles"(page 71)	*Keto Margherit-o Pizza*
Keto Margherit-o Pizza	*Avocado "Fries"*	Vegan Niçoise Salad (page 95) Italian Wedding Soup (page 111)

WEEK 2 SHOPPING LIST

FATS AND OILS

- Almond butter (4¼ cups)
- Chia seeds (⅝ cup)
- Coconut flakes, unsweetened (4 cups)
- Coconut oil (½ cup)
- Flaxseed, ground (2 tablespoons)
- Hemp seeds (1¾ cups)
- MCT oil (3 tablespoons)
- Cold-pressed olive oil (6⅝ cups)
- Pine nuts, dried (½ cup)
- Walnuts, raw (4 cups)

PRODUCE

- Arugula (1 [5-ounce]) bag
- Avocados (5)
- Basil, fresh (2 bunches)
- Broccoli, florets (1 pound)
- Butter leaf lettuce (2 heads)
- Butternut squash (1)
- Carrots (1 bundle)
- Cauliflower (2 large heads)
- Celery (1 bunch)
- Chives (1 bunch)
- Daikon radish (1)
- Garlic (4 cloves)
- Ginger root, fresh (1 large piece)
- Grapefruit (1 medium)
- Green beans (1 pound)
- Green peas, frozen (2 cups)
- Leeks (2)
- Lettuce (1 head)
- Lettuce, romaine (1 head)
- Lemongrass
- Lemons (12)
- Mint, fresh (1 bunch)
- Mushrooms (3 [10-ounce]) boxes
- Scallions (1 bunch)

- Onions, red (3)
- Parsley, fresh (3 bunches)
- Bell peppers, green (5)
- Bell peppers, yellow (1)
- Radishes (5)
- Raspberries (1 [8-ounce]) container
- Shallots (2)
- Spinach (6 pounds)
- Thyme, fresh
- Tomatoes, cherry (4¼ cups)
- Tomatoes, heirloom (4 pounds)
- Tomatoes, Roma (6)
- Zucchini, large (2)

PANTRY ITEMS (brands we like are in parentheses)

- Almond flour
- Cold-brew coffee (Bulletproof, Chameleon, or Four Sigmatic)
- Cacao powder
- Coconut cream
- Coconut milk, full-fat
- Coconut flour
- Liquid smoke, hickory
- Liquid stevia (Omica, Sweetleaf, or NuNaturals)
- Marsala wine, dry
- Miso paste
- Monk fruit sweetener (Lakanto or You Are Loved Foods)
- Mushroom broth (Pacific Foods)
- Olives, black sliced
- Psyllium husks
- Soybeans, black
- Maple-flavored syrup (Lakanto or NuNaturals)
- Tahini
- Tamari
- Stewed tomatoes
- Tomato paste
- Tomato sauce
- Vegetable broth (Pacific Foods)
- Vinegar, white
- Vinegar, apple cider

DRIED HERBS, SPICES, AND BAKING INGREDIENTS

- Bay leaves (5)
- Black peppercorns
- Cardamom, ground
- Cayenne pepper
- Cinnamon, ground
- Coriander seeds
- Cumin seeds
- Garlic powder
- Mint, dried
- Nutritional yeast seasoning (Bragg, Pop Zest, or Noochy Licious by Gloriously Vegan)
- Oregano, dried
- Paprika
- Red pepper flakes
- Sea salt
- Vanilla extract

ABOUT THESE RECIPES

You don't need a lot of cooking experience to prepare the recipes in this book. They were all designed to be simple, fast, and budget-friendly. We've done our best to avoid hard-to-find ingredients, but you may see some unfamiliar items that you'll soon get to know and enjoy.

Since this book is about the vegan keto diet, all recipes are plant-based and contain no animal fats or proteins. They're also gluten-free and low soy, and most of the nuts in the recipes can be swapped for seeds (see the tips for substitutions).

We've done the nutritional calculations for you, including the macro ratios, so you can enjoy each dish without worrying if it's keto. However, we encourage you to follow the serving sizes and be mindful about the net carbs in relation to what else you ate and plan to eat for the day. You'll see a handful of recipes with net carbs of 21 grams or higher—five in total. Please be mindful of these as you're working toward ketosis. The higher carb meals are best after you've stabilized your ketosis and want to treat yourself with a more hearty meal. The recipes are filling, nutritious, and delicious, to keep you feeling nourished and satisfied.

QUICK RECIPES FOR FLAX "EGGS" AND CAULIFLOWER "RICE"

A few of our recipes call for a flax "egg" and riced cauliflower. Here's a quick tutorial on how to make them.

- To make a flax "egg," combine 1 tablespoon of ground flax-seed meal with 3 tablespoons of water. After about 5 minutes the mixture will have a thick, sticky consistency and will be ready to be used in place of eggs in baked goods.

- You can purchase pre-made riced cauliflower (sometimes labeled as cauliflower rice) in the refrigerated produce and frozen sections of many grocery stores. But if you prefer to make your own, simply put cauliflower florets in a food processor and pulse until they form rice-like shapes.

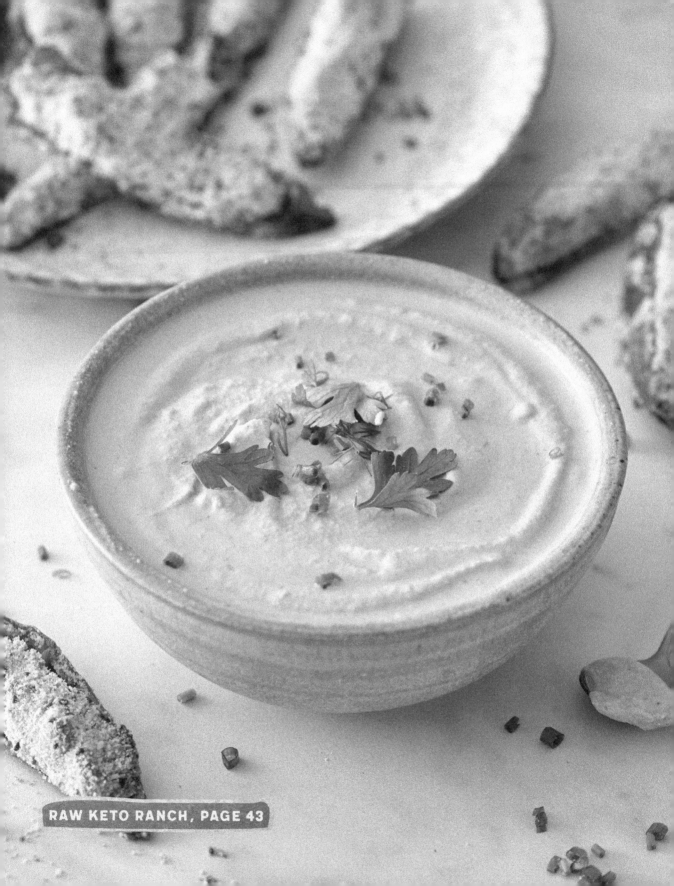

RAW KETO RANCH, PAGE 43

SAUCES & DRESSINGS

Don't let anyone tell you that plant-based food is boring! Sauces and dressings add pizzazz and make everything taste incredible. Whenever you want to spruce up a plate of veggies, add a sauce or dressing to transform them. For example, cauliflower is delicious on its own and gets ramped up to another level when covered with vegan nacho cheese. The following recipes feature classic flavors from America, Europe, and Asia to ensure that you don't miss out on your favorite foods.

CHIMICHURRI SAUCE

This sauce originates from Argentina, where it is pretty much a mandatory accompaniment to meat. It's also fabulous with other dishes and good for you. It is loaded with parsley and cilantro that help with the detoxification of heavy metals while giving you a plant-happy boost of chlorophyll.

1 cup cold-pressed olive oil	¼ cup fresh mint	1 garlic clove
½ cup fresh parsley	1 tablespoon dried oregano	1 shallot
⅓ cup fresh cilantro		Juice of 1 lemon

1. Put all the ingredients into a high-powered blender and pulse until well combined and a bit chunky.
2. Store the chimichurri in a covered container in the refrigerator for up to 1 week. Smear it on everything savory for a flavorful snack or to liven up a meal.

COOKING TIP: *To add a surprising and tangy twist to this sauce, add 2 tablespoons of capers. Try it with Market Veggie Tofu Scramble (page 66).*

Per Serving: Calories: 164; Total fat: 18g; Carbohydrates: 1g; Fiber: <1g; Net carbs: 1g; Protein: <1g.

RAW KETO RANCH

Who said following a diet plan means missing out on the foods you love? You can still have ranch. This dressing has a healthy dose of apple cider vinegar to help alkalize your body. Dr. Otto Warburg said, "No disease, including cancer, can exist in an alkaline environment." So, go ahead and bust out your favorite veggies and get dipping.

1 cup raw cashews, soaked overnight

½ cup water

2 teaspoons apple cider vinegar

1½ teaspoons freshly squeezed lemon juice

2 tablespoons finely chopped fresh dill

2 tablespoons finely chopped fresh chives

1 tablespoon finely chopped fresh Italian parsley

¼ teaspoon sea salt

¼ teaspoon onion powder

¼ teaspoon garlic powder

In a food processor or bullet blender, combine all the ingredients and blend on high until a creamy consistency is reached.

COOKING TIP: *To make this a dip, use half the amount of water for a thicker texture. The dip is great with broccoli florets and celery, and makes a crunchy, high-fiber snack.*

Per Serving: Calories: 61; Total fat: 5g; Carbohydrates: 3g; Fiber: 1g; Net carbs: 2g; Protein: 2g

THAI-STYLE PEANUT SAUCE

SERVES 6 · PREP TIME: 5 MINUTES

This satisfying sauce is a perfect go-to when hunger hits and you need to whip up something quickly. Peanuts are a great source of fat and protein, which offer sustained energy. You can put this sauce on just about anything to make it feel like a treat.

½ cup sugar-free peanut butter

1 tablespoon miso paste

1 shallot, peeled

3 tablespoons peeled and finely chopped fresh ginger

1 teaspoon sesame oil

⅓ cup freshly squeezed lime juice

2 tablespoons monk fruit sweetener

¼ cup lightly crushed peanuts, for garnish

1. Combine all the ingredients except crushed peanuts in a high-powered blender and blend for about 3 minutes.
2. For a silkier texture, slowly add a few tablespoons of water while blending.
3. Transfer the sauce to an airtight container and store in the refrigerator until ready to use.

INGREDIENT TIP: *Garnish with freshly crushed peanuts before serving, to add a fun texture.*

SUBSTITUTION TIP: *Tahini paste can be substituted for the peanut butter, and sesame seeds for the peanuts, in case of peanut allergies.*

Per Serving: Calories: 181; Total fat: 15g; Carbohydrates: 9g; Fiber: 2g; Net carbs: 7g; Protein: 7g

"NACHO CHEESE" SAUCE

SERVES 6 · PREP TIME: 10 MINUTES, PLUS OVERNIGHT SOAKING ·
COOK TIME: 35 MINUTES

If you're wondering how to do vegan keto and still enjoy nacho cheese sauce, we've got the answer. This upgraded version is high in protein and healthy fats to keep you feeling satisfied. Whip up a batch and have it at the ready for your next Netflix binge.

½ head cauliflower, broken into florets

1 cup peeled and coarsely chopped butternut squash

2 cups vegetable broth, divided

1 cup almonds, soaked overnight

⅓ cup nutritional yeast

1 teaspoon sea salt

1 teaspoon freshly ground black pepper

2 teaspoons paprika

½ jalapeño pepper (optional)

1 tablespoon apple cider vinegar

1. Bring a large pot of water to a boil over medium-high heat. Add the cauliflower and butternut squash to the pot, reduce the heat to medium, and cook until completely tender, about 25 minutes.
2. Strain the vegetables and set them aside.
3. In a high-powered blender, combine 1 cup of broth, the almonds, nutritional yeast, salt, pepper, paprika, jalapeño (if using), and apple cider vinegar. Blend until smooth.
4. Slowly add the cauliflower and squash, blending as you go. Once the vegetables have been added, pulse until a smooth, thick, cheese-like consistency is reached.
5. Store in the refrigerator until ready to serve.

LEFTOVERS TIP: *For a warm nacho cheese, you can simply reheat the sauce in a small saucepan and serve over flax crackers to create keto nachos, or pour it over broccoli for a satisfying snack.*

STORAGE TIP: *Keep in an airtight container in the refrigerator for up to 1 week. Do not freeze.*

Per Serving: Calories: 181; Total fat: 12g; Carbohydrates: 14g; Fiber: 6g; Net carbs: 8g; Protein: 9g

VEGAN "SOUR CREAM"

SERVES 12 · PREP TIME: 5 MINUTES, PLUS OVERNIGHT
SOAKING AND A SECOND NIGHT TO FERMENT

Our vegan keto eating plan is not about missing out on favorite foods; it's about making upgrades to old classics and living life to its fullest. This "sour cream" is naturally fermented to add a probiotic boost and support healthy gut flora without the negative environmental impacts of consuming dairy.

1 cup raw almonds, soaked overnight

Juice of ½ lemon

1 teaspoon nutritional yeast

⅓ teaspoon sea salt

¼ cup water, plus more if needed

1. Put the soaked almonds in a high-powered blender with the lemon juice, nutritional yeast, salt, and water, and blend until creamy and smooth. Add more water if necessary.

2. Spoon the mixture into an airtight container and place in a cool, dark cabinet to allow the cream to ferment overnight. This fermentation is what gives the cream that tart "sour cream" flavor.

3. In the morning, place the mixture in the refrigerator to store until needed. It will last for up to 1 week.

COOKING TIP: *To make a sweet cream topping for desserts or berries, omit the nutritional yeast, and add 4 or 5 drops of liquid stevia and a teaspoon of ground cinnamon. Mix it together, and use it to top any dessert.*

Per Serving: Calories: 66; Total fat: 6g; Carbohydrates: 3g; Fiber: 1g; Net carbs: 2g; Protein: 3g

HERB GARDEN DRESSING

SERVES 12 · PREP TIME: 5 MINUTES

There's a well-known bakery in downtown Los Angeles that many people in the city attest has the best salad dressing. Nicole ordered this salad for a week straight until she figured out how to recreate the dressing at home. You're welcome. You can make this dressing on the weekend to have it on hand for easy salad prep during the week.

1 cup cold-pressed olive oil	¼ cup fresh dill	1 shallot
Juice of 3 lemons	¼ cup fresh parsley	Sea salt
¼ cup fresh mint	¼ cup fresh cilantro	Freshly ground black pepper
	¼ cup fresh tarragon	

1. Combine all the ingredients in a high-powered blender and blend until thoroughly amalgamated and smooth.
2. Store the dressing in a covered container in the refrigerator for up to 1 week.

COOKING TIP: *To turn this into more of a dip, add 1 cup of cauliflower rice or raw almonds and blend with the rest of the ingredients. This will create a thicker texture as well as provide a fiber boost for sustained satisfaction.*

Per Serving: Calories: 165; Total fat: 18g; Carbohydrates: 1g; Fiber: <1g; Net carbs: 1g; Protein: <1g

GINGER-LIME DRESSING

The ginger and lime in this dressing create a perfect marriage of flavors. What's more, the citrus juice will boost your immune system and support healthy heart function, and the fresh ginger will warm your body, reduce inflammation, and get your blood pumping.

1 cup cold-pressed olive oil

Juice of 3 limes

2 inches fresh ginger, peeled

1 teaspoon ground cumin

⅓ teaspoon ground cardamom

1 drop liquid stevia

Sea salt

1. Combine all the ingredients in a high-powered blender and blend on high until thoroughly amalgamated and smooth.
2. Store the dressing in a covered container in the refrigerator for up to 1 week.

COOKING TIP: *To boost the anti-inflammatory properties of this dressing, add 2 teaspoons of dried turmeric. This will also give the dressing a bright and beautiful color.*

Per Serving: Calories: 245; Total fat: 27g; Carbohydrates: <1g; Fiber: <1g; Net carbs: 0g; Protein: <1g

TAHINI GODDESS

Tahini, a Middle Eastern paste made with sesame seeds, is often used to flavor hummus and baba ghanoush. It is highly nutritious and can help prevent brittle bones through boosting bone cell growth. The healthy fats contained in tahini also support optimal brain function.

Juice of 1 large or
2 small lemons

3 tablespoons raw tahini

¼ cup water

½ teaspoon
smoked paprika

⅛ teaspoon cayenne
pepper (optional)

Freshly ground
black pepper

Sea salt

1. In a medium bowl, whisk the lemon juice, tahini, and water until well blended.
2. Add the paprika and cayenne (if using), and season with salt and pepper. Mix until well combined.
3. Keep the dressing in a covered container in the pantry for up to 6 months. In the refrigerator, it will last for up to 1 year.

COOKING TIP: *If a less tart flavor is preferred, add a drop or two of liquid stevia to offset the lemon juice.*

Per Serving: Calories: 40; Total fat: 3g; Carbohydrates: 2g; Fiber: 1g; Net carbs: 1g; Protein: 1g

RAW PESTO

The first time Nicole ate pesto from scratch it was after her uncle trimmed a few handfuls of fresh basil from a bush in his backyard. A few minutes later she was eating one of the best meals of her life. Nicole was amazed at how simple it is to make fresh pesto and she is excited to share this adaptation of her family recipe with you. Walnuts have been added to replace Parmesan cheese and add a cancer-fighting boost.

4 garlic cloves	4 cups fresh basil leaves	2 teaspoons sea salt
1 cup cold-pressed olive oil	½ cup freshly squeezed lemon juice	⅓ cup raw walnuts

1. In a food processor, pulse together the garlic and olive oil until roughly chopped.
2. Add the basil, lemon juice, and salt.
3. Blend until creamy, about 3 minutes. Add the walnuts and pulse until your desired texture is achieved.

COOKING TIP: *A smoother texture is better for a sauce. A thicker and chunkier texture is better for dipping.*

STORAGE TIP: *Store in an airtight jar and keep in the refrigerator for up to 1 week.*

Per Serving: Calories: 377; Total fat: 41g; Carbohydrates: 4g; Fiber: 2g; Net carbs: 2g; Protein: 2g

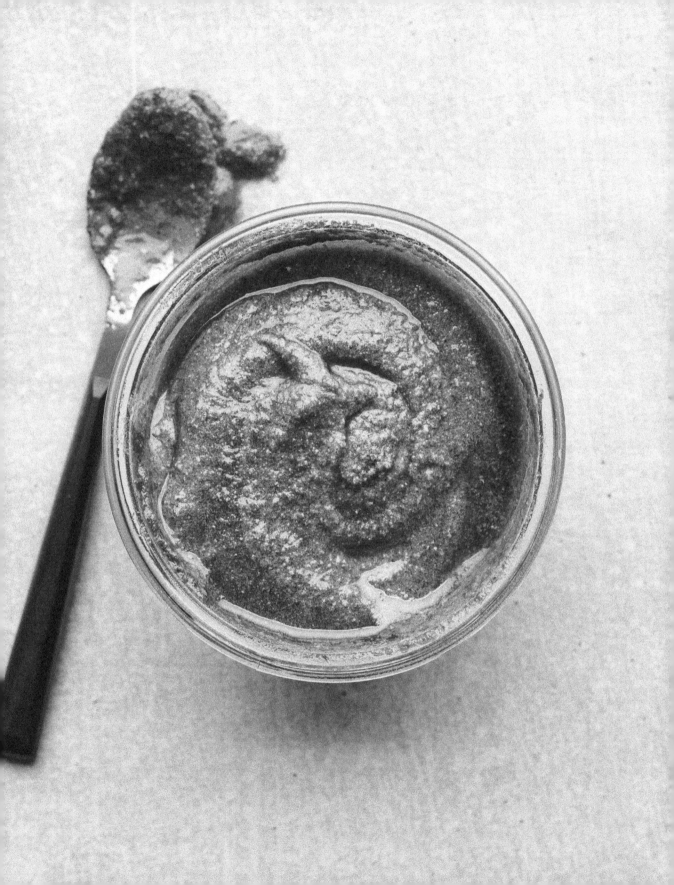

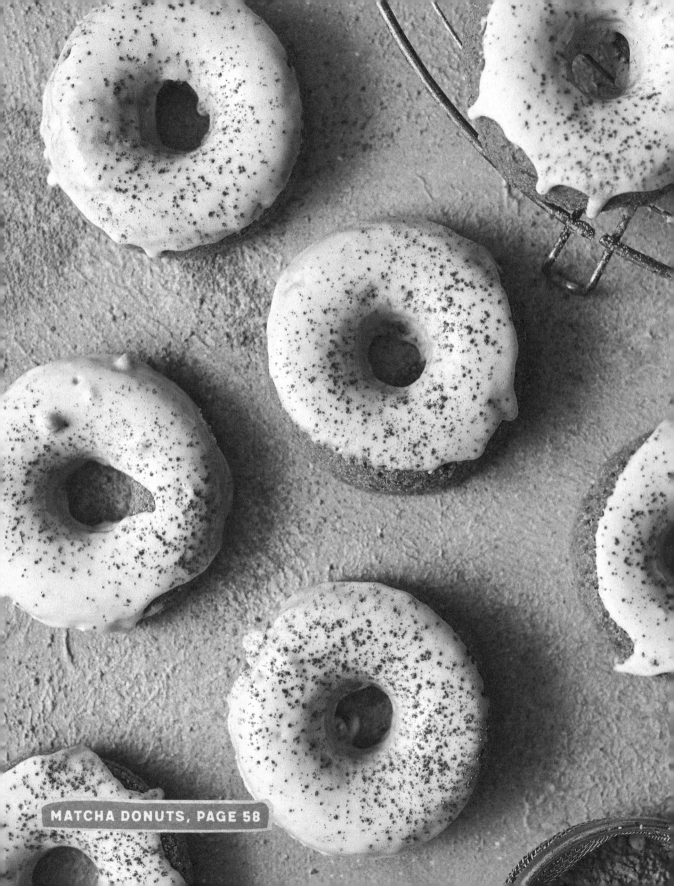

MATCHA DONUTS, PAGE 58

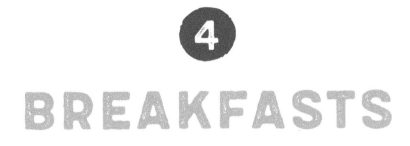

BREAKFASTS

Unless you're intermittent fasting and skipping breakfast, there's no reason you can't enjoy pancakes and donuts while on the vegan keto diet. We're thrilled to present low-carb, plant-based versions of the classics. We have scrambled "eggs," quiche, and breakfast tostadas. Want a smoothie without the sugar? There are two to choose from here, plus a keto take on overnight oats and avocado toast. Next time someone offers to make you breakfast in bed, hand them this book with this chapter bookmarked.

COFFEE SMOOTHIE

SERVES 2 · PREP TIME: 5 MINUTES

Can't talk before your first cup of coffee of the day? Here is your coffee and breakfast all in one. The caffeine in this recipe will give you a wake-up boost while the fats from the avocado fuel your brain and prevent your body crashing before lunch time. Enjoy your superpowers.

1 cup unsweetened hemp milk

½ cup ice

⅓ cup cold-brew coffee

½ avocado

2 tablespoons cacao powder

1 scoop plant-based, low-carb protein powder (such as Truvani or Sunwarrior brands) (optional)

2 or 3 drops liquid stevia

1. Combine all the ingredients in a blender and blend on high until creamy and smooth.
2. Divide between tall serving glasses and enjoy chilled.

COOKING TIP: *If you are an ardent coffee lover, add a tablespoon of coffee grounds to this smoothie to amp up the flavor even more, without watering down the texture.*

Per Serving: Calories: 130; Total fat: 9g; Carbohydrates: 8g; Fiber: 4g; Net carbs: 4g; Protein: 3g

CHIA PARFAIT

SERVES 4 · PREP TIME: 5 MINUTES, PLUS AT LEAST 20 MINUTES TO CHILL

Talk about a power breakfast; this parfait will leave you feeling satisfied for hours. Chia seeds are extraordinarily potent sources of antioxidants and fiber. The almond milk gives you protein, and the coconut cream provides fat. And did we mention how good it tastes?

2½ cups unsweetened almond milk

½ cup coconut cream

1 teaspoon ground cinnamon

¼ teaspoon ground cardamom

⅛ teaspoon ground nutmeg

1 teaspoon vanilla extract

¼ cup chia seeds

1. Pour the almond milk and coconut cream into a 32-ounce mason jar.
2. Add the cinnamon, cardamom, nutmeg, vanilla, and chia seeds.
3. Close the lid tightly and shake the jar vigorously.
4. Place the jar in the refrigerator to set for at least 20 minutes or overnight.

INGREDIENT TIP: *Top the parfait with berries for an antioxidant boost, or add your favorite plant-based, low-carb protein powder for sustained energy on active days.*

Per Serving: Calories: 150; Total fat: 11g; Carbohydrates: 8g; Fiber: 6g; Net carbs: 2g; Protein: 4g

PB&J OVERNIGHT HEMP

SERVES 6 · PREP TIME: 5 MINUTES, PLUS OVERNIGHT TO SET

This recipe might make you feel like a kid again, but your grown-up self will know that your breakfast is full of fiber and great for sustained energy to get you through busy mornings. It's one breakfast you definitely won't want to trade with your friends. The hemp hearts contain arginine, an amino acid that helps prevent heart disease.

3 cups unsweetened almond milk, plus more for serving

1 tablespoon sugar-free peanut butter

4 drops liquid stevia or sugar-free sweetener of choice

1½ cups hemp hearts

2 tablespoons chia seeds

¼ cup cacao nibs

⅛ cup unsweetened coconut flakes

¼ cup freeze-dried raspberries

1. In a large mixing bowl, whisk together the almond milk, peanut butter, and stevia.

2. Once well combined, add the hemp hearts, chia seeds, cacao nibs, coconut, and raspberries, and stir together.

3. Pour the mixture into a lidded storage container and place in the refrigerator for at least 8 hours.

4. Divide the mixture among 6 small serving bowls and top with a splash of almond milk.

SUBSTITUTION TIP: *Swap out the peanut butter for almond butter or tahini to accommodate nut allergies.*

Per Serving: Calories: 324; Total fat: 24g; Carbohydrates: 10g; Fiber: 8g; Net carbs: 2g; Protein: 16g

GO GET 'EM GREEN SMOOTHIE BOWL

SERVES 2 · PREP TIME: 5 MINUTES

Smoothie bowls can be especially appealing in hot and humid weather when you might not feel like cooking. They are easy ways to get a whole lot of nutrients in a tasty package. The MCT in this recipe helps boost energy, increase brain function, and lower cholesterol. The spinach is rich in vitamins A and C, the avocado gives you a hit of monounsaturated fat, the almond milk and butter are nutritional powerhouses, and the ginger provides a healthy kick.

2 cups fresh spinach

1 cup unsweetened almond milk

½ cup ice cubes

½ avocado

1 tablespoon MCT oil

1 tablespoon almond butter

1 handful fresh mint leaves

4 drops liquid stevia

½-inch fresh ginger, peeled

Optional toppings:

Hemp or chia seeds

Coconut flakes

Cacao nibs

Fresh mint

Sliced strawberries

1. Combine the spinach, almond milk, ice, avocado, MCT oil, almond butter, mint, stevia, and ginger in a high-powered blender. Blend on high until smooth and thick, adding a little extra liquid if needed.

2. Scoop the smoothie mixture into a bowl and sprinkle with your choice of toppings.

INGREDIENT TIP: *Buy fresh spinach from the farmers' market or the organic section of the grocery store. Store spinach in the freezer to keep it fresh and on hand.*

Per Serving: Calories: 214; Total fat: 20g; Carbohydrates: 8g; Fiber: 5g; Net carbs: 3g; Protein: 3g

MATCHA DONUTS

SERVES 6 • PREP TIME: 10 MINUTES • COOK TIME: 13 MINUTES

Matcha was developed in China, then brought to Japan, where it became popular in monastic society and then spread to military and upper-class use. Green tea leaves were ground into a fine concentrated powder that the warriors could carry easily and mix with river water to replenish their bodies. You can gain the same benefit by sprinkling that matcha magic into your keto donuts.

FOR THE DONUTS

Nonstick coconut oil cooking spray

2 cups almond flour

⅓ cup powdered stevia

1½ tablespoons matcha powder

1 tablespoon baking powder

¼ teaspoon salt

¾ cup unsweetened hemp or almond milk

2 tablespoons freshly squeezed lemon juice

1 teaspoon vanilla extract

1 flax "egg" (see page 39)

6 tablespoons tahini

FOR THE ICING

¼ cup coconut oil

¼ cup powdered stevia

1 teaspoon vanilla extract

½ teaspoon matcha powder

TO MAKE THE DONUTS

1. Preheat the oven to 350°F. Grease a donut pan with cooking spray and set aside.
2. In a large mixing bowl, whisk together the almond flour, stevia, matcha powder, baking powder, and salt.
3. In a separate mixing bowl, whisk together the hemp milk, lemon juice, vanilla, flax "egg," and tahini.
4. Pour the wet mixture into the dry mixture and stir gently to combine. Do not overwork the batter.

5. Fill the prepared donut pan with the batter, and bake for 13 minutes.

6. Remove the pan from the oven and poke a donut with a toothpick to check for doneness. If the toothpick is clean when you remove it, set the donuts, still in the pan, on a rack to cool for about 15 minutes. (Removing them from the pan fresh out of the oven can cause them to break.)

TO MAKE THE ICING

1. In a small mixing bowl, combine the coconut oil, stevia, vanilla, and matcha. Whisk until thoroughly blended.

2. Dip the top of the donuts into the icing and sprinkle with Matcha powder, if desired, and serve while still slightly warm.

COOKING TIP: *If you don't have a donut pan, this recipe works great as a Bundt cake. Don't forget to spray your Bundt pan with nonstick cooking spray.*

Per Serving: Calories: 296; Total fat: 28g; Carbohydrates: 9g; Fiber: 5g; Net carbs: 4g; Protein: 8g

ALMOND AND VANILLA PANCAKES

SERVES 4 · PREP TIME: 10 MINUTES · COOK TIME: 15 MINUTES

Nicole's mom used to make a special pancake breakfast on Sunday mornings. Just say the word "pancakes" and Nicole's heart floods with warm memories of waking up at the family home. To keep that memory alive, she created this version which is high in good-for-you ingredients that will comfort you and fill you up. Make this dish on the weekend or when you are in need of a little love.

⅔ cup unsweetened almond milk

1 tablespoon apple cider vinegar

4 tablespoons coconut oil or vegan butter

1 teaspoon vanilla extract

1 cup coconut flour

1 cup almond flour

2 tablespoons ground flaxseed

½ teaspoon baking powder

Coconut oil cooking spray

Almond slivers, for serving

Vegan butter or coconut oil, for serving

Sugar-free maple syrup for topping

1. Preheat the oven to a warming setting.
2. Combine the almond milk, vinegar, coconut oil, and vanilla in a high-powered blender and blend until thoroughly amalgamated.
3. Add the coconut flour, almond flour, flaxseed, and baking powder. Blend for 3 full minutes until the batter is full and fluffy. If the batter seems too thick, slowly add a few tablespoons of water to thin it out. Set the mixture aside.
4. Heat a medium skillet over medium-low heat and coat it with coconut oil spray to prevent sticking.

5. Once the skillet is hot, pour a small portion of batter into the pan, and cook for about 3 minutes (or until the top of the batter stops bubbling).

6. Flip the pancake and cook until toasted on the opposite side.

7. Place the finished pancake on a warming rack in the oven to keep warm.

8. Repeat steps 5 to 7 until all of the batter has been cooked.

9. Top the pancakes with almond slivers and vegan butter. Drizzle with the maple syrup and serve.

STORAGE TIP: *The batter can be made in advance and stored in the refrigerator for up to 1 week. Keep it in an airtight container or, even better, a squeeze bottle. You can squeeze batter directly out of the bottle into the hot skillet. Don't forget to shake the bottle first, because the batter will separate.*

Per Serving: Calories: 426; Total fat: 33g; Carbohydrates: 28g; Fiber: 16g; Net carbs: 12g; Protein: 11g

AVOCADO BOATS *with* FLAX CRACKERS

SERVES 2 · PREP TIME: 10 MINUTES

This recipe is a keto adaptation of Nicole's favorite breakfast at her favorite spot in Hollywood. Avocado is rich in monounsaturated omega-9, and flax seeds provide lots of fiber and omega-3s to help lower the risk of heart disease, cancer, and diabetes.

1 Roma tomato, chopped

2 tablespoons cold-pressed olive oil, plus more for drizzling

1 tablespoon fresh basil, plus more, cut into chiffonade, for serving

1 garlic clove, crushed

Sea salt

⅛ teaspoon freshly ground black pepper

1 avocado, halved and pit removed

Juice of ½ lemon

Flaxseed crackers

1. In a small mixing bowl, gently toss the tomato, olive oil, basil, garlic, salt, and pepper, and set aside.
2. Sprinkle the cut surface of the avocado halves with the lemon juice to prevent browning.
3. Generously stuff the avocado halves with the tomato mixture.
4. Plate the stuffed avocado, drizzle with olive oil, and top with a few ribbons of fresh basil.
5. Serve with flax crackers.

INGREDIENT TIP: *To enjoy perfectly ripe avocado for this dish, buy the avocados a few days beforehand and put them in a brown bag to ripen. For extremely firm avocados, add a ripe banana to the bag, which will speed up the ripening process.*

Per Serving: Calories: 286; Total fat: 28g; Carbohydrates: 12g; Fiber: 7g; Net carbs: 5g; Protein: 2g

BREAKFAST TOSTADAS

SERVES 2 · PREP TIME: 10 MINUTES · COOK TIME: 10 MINUTES

When Nicole was a kid, her family spent each Thanksgiving in San Felipe, Mexico. She remembers mornings on the Baja coast with her siblings, with ocean mist blasting their faces. This dish, inspired by those vacations, is as fun as it is hydrating and full of healthy enzymes. The net carbs here equal 22 grams, so keep this in mind as you plan your meals for the day.

1 peeled jicama

1 tablespoon coconut oil

3 cups cauliflower rice

1 teaspoon ground paprika

1 teaspoon ground coriander

1 teaspoon ground oregano

½ teaspoon ground cumin

1 avocado, sliced

⅓ cup pico de gallo or fresh salsa, divided

¼ cup Vegan "Sour Cream" (page 46)

¼ cup chopped fresh cilantro

1. Using a mandoline or a chef's knife, slice the jicama into thin discs and set aside.

2. Warm the coconut oil in a large skillet over medium heat. Toss in the cauliflower rice, paprika, coriander, oregano, and cumin.

3. Cook, stirring often and allowing any excess water to cook off, for about 6 minutes.

4. Once the cauliflower starts to become tender, remove the skillet from the heat.

5. To make the tostadas, place the jicama slices on a platter.

6. On top of the disks, spoon the cauliflower, avocado, pico de gallo, "sour cream," and cilantro.

LEFTOVERS TIP: *Extra jicama can be cut into sticks and saved for dipping or munching by itself between meals. It tastes great with freshly squeezed lime juice or dipped into Raw Keto Ranch (page 43).*

Per Serving: Calories: 479; Total fat: 30g; Carbohydrates: 51g; Fiber: 29g; Net carbs: 22g; Protein: 13g

TUSCAN "QUICHE" BITES

SERVES 4 · PREP TIME: 15 MINUTES · COOK TIME: 45 MINUTES

These "quiches" are a satisfying crowd pleaser. They are also the perfect make-ahead dish for weekly meal prep or your next potluck. Loaded with protein from the tofu, these bites keep you energized and moving. Nutritional yeast, which adds a great cheesy flavor, makes the dish high in B vitamins 1, 2, 3, 6, and 12. It also helps re-mineralize the body.

2 tablespoons cold-pressed olive oil

½ cup sliced cremini mushrooms

⅓ cup chopped onion

¼ cup sliced cherry tomatoes

1 teaspoon garlic powder

1 cup coarsely chopped fresh spinach

¼ cup sliced black olives

1 (14-ounce) block organic firm sprouted tofu, drained

¼ cup water

2 tablespoons tahini

2 tablespoons nutritional yeast

1 teaspoon dried basil

1 teaspoon dried oregano

¼ teaspoon ground cumin

⅛ teaspoon turmeric powder

½ teaspoon kala namak salt (optional; see Tip)

Nonstick cooking spray

1. Preheat the oven to 350°F.
2. Heat the olive oil in a large skillet over medium heat. Add the mushrooms, onion, tomatoes, and garlic powder, and sauté for about 5 minutes. Once the mushrooms start to sweat and the tomatoes start to blister, turn off the heat.
3. Stir in the spinach and olives and set aside.
4. In a blender, combine the tofu with the water, tahini, nutritional yeast, basil, oregano, cumin, turmeric, and salt (if using). Blend until a fluffy, egglike consistency is obtained, adding a little more water if needed.

5. Transfer the mixture to a large mixing bowl and fold in the sautéed vegetables.

6. Coat a six-cup muffin pan with cooking spray. Divide the batter equally among the muffin cups.

7. Bake in the preheated oven for 45 minutes until a toothpick inserted into the center of a quiche comes out clean.

8. Allow the quiches to cool for 10 minutes before serving, because the centers will be very hot.

COOKING TIP: *Top with Raw Pesto (page 50) and fresh basil for a real wow factor. Pesto will make all the flavors really pop, while adding an antioxidant boost.*

INGREDIENT TIP: *Kala namak is a volcanic salt with a sulfuric flavor, reminiscent of egg yolk. If you have trouble finding it or don't want to purchase an additional seasoning, just leave it out.*

Per Serving: Calories: 241; Total fat: 18g; Carbohydrates: 7g; Fiber: 3g; Net carbs: 4g; Protein: 14g

MARKET VEGGIE TOFU SCRAMBLE

SERVES 4 · PREP TIME: 10 MINUTES · COOK TIME: 10 MINUTES

This a riff on that '90s vegan classic: the tofu scramble. In southern California there are countless spots that serve up the plant-based breakfast staple, so we know what it takes to make the best one. Nicole revised her own version time and again to present you with the perfect tofu scramble.

1 (14-ounce) block firm sprouted organic tofu, pressed and drained

2 tablespoons tahini

2 tablespoons nutritional yeast

1 tablespoon chia seeds

¼ teaspoon turmeric powder

⅛ teaspoon kala namak salt

2 tablespoons cold-pressed coconut oil

⅓ cup diced yellow onion

⅓ cup diced green bell pepper

¼ teaspoon garlic powder

¼ cup olives

2 cups coarsely chopped fresh spinach

1 teaspoon hot sauce (optional)

1. Blot the tofu with a paper towel to remove as much water as possible, then crumble it by hand into a large mixing bowl.
2. Add the tahini, nutritional yeast, chia seeds, turmeric, and kala namak salt to the bowl. Toss the ingredients together and set aside.
3. Heat the coconut oil in a large skillet over medium heat.
4. Add the onion, bell pepper, and garlic powder to the skillet.
5. Once the vegetables are tender and caramelized, toss in the olives and tofu mixture.

6. Allow the tofu to cook undisturbed for about 4 minutes to create a toasted, hash-like texture, then toss once to toast it a bit more.

7. Once the tofu is toasty, remove the skillet from the heat and stir in the spinach until it wilts.

8. Serve with your favorite hot sauce (if using).

MAKE-AHEAD TIP: *For faster meal prep, prepare the tofu in advance by draining, crumbling, and mixing it with the tahini, nutritional yeast, chia seeds, turmeric, and salt. The tofu will absorb more flavor this way, and prepping the dish in advance will be faster for a midweek breakfast. The prepared mixture can be kept in the refrigerator for up to 1 week.*

Per Serving: Calories: 253; Total fat: 18g; Carbohydrates: 11g; Fiber: 4g; Net carbs: 7g; Protein: 15g

JALEPEÑO POPPERS, PAGE 72

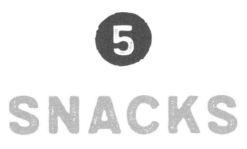

SNACKS

If you're anything like us, you love snacking. Sometimes it's about satisfying a craving for something sweet; other times there's an intense desire for a savory crunch, and at times you just need a little something between meals. On the vegan keto diet, you might want to up your calorie intake, or you may need a little more to fulfill your daily macro ratio. No matter why you want a snack, we have 11 recipes to hit the spot.

ZUCCHINI CHIPS

SERVES 6 · PREP TIME: 10 MINUTES · COOK TIME: 2 HOURS

Salty and crunchy, these zucchini chips are light yet satisfying and a great go-to when hunger strikes. They're especially handy when you don't want to go over your macros for the day. Don't let the simplicity of this recipe fool you, either; the chips are a good source of vitamins C and A, thiamin, niacin, and fiber.

1 large zucchini, cut into thin disks	1 teaspoon sea salt	1 teaspoon dried dill
	2 tablespoons coconut oil	1 tablespoon freshly ground black pepper

1. Preheat the oven to 225°F.
2. Line a baking sheet with parchment paper. If you don't have parchment paper, use aluminum foil or a greased pan.
3. Sprinkle the zucchini slices with the salt and spread them out on paper towels.
4. With a separate paper towel, firmly press the zucchini slices and pat them dry (the dryer the better).
5. Toss the zucchini slices in the coconut oil, dill, and pepper, then spread them out on the prepared baking sheet.
6. Bake for 2 hours, or until they are golden and crisp. Check every 30 minutes or so for burn marks. If you begin to see them burn, remove the chips immediately.
7. Remove the chips from the oven and cool.
8. Once the chips have cooled, transfer them to a serving bowl or store in an airtight container for up to 3 days.

COOKING TIP: *To create barbecue chips, toss the slices in your favorite barbecue rub and a few drops of liquid stevia before baking. Be sure not to oversalt them.*

Per Serving: Calories: 52; Total fat: 5g; Carbohydrates: 3g; Fiber: 1g; Net carbs: 1g; Protein: 1g

TURMERIC CAULIFLOWER "PICKLES"

SERVES 6 · PREP TIME: 10 MINUTES ·
COOK TIME: 5 MINUTES, PLUS 3 DAYS TO FERMENT

These satisfyingly crunchy pickles check off the anti-inflammatory requirement that many of us search for when we eat. These beauties are amazing snacks on their own and have the power to make any dish pop. Plus, the turmeric adds a brilliant and beautiful color to the cauliflower.

1 cauliflower head, cut into florets	½ cup powdered monk fruit sweetener	1 teaspoon turmeric powder
⅔ cup white vinegar	1 tablespoon sea salt	1 bay leaf
⅓ cup water	1 teaspoon ground coriander	1 teaspoon peppercorns

1. Place the cauliflower florets in large Mason jars.
2. In a medium saucepan over medium heat, combine the vinegar, water, monk fruit sweetener, salt, coriander, turmeric, bay leaf, and peppercorns. Bring the brine to a low simmer for 5 minutes. Remove the pan from the heat and allow it to cool.
3. Once the brine has cooled, pour it over the cauliflower in the jars.
4. Be sure to fill the jars all the way to the top to ensure that the cauliflower is completely covered.
5. Close the jars to make them as airtight as possible.
6. Store the jars in the refrigerator for 3 days to ferment before eating.

INGREDIENT TIP: *Enjoy as a snack or toss into your next salad for extra flair. The pickles will keep in the refrigerator for over a month.*

Per Serving: Calories: 26; Total fat: <1g; Carbohydrates: 5g; Fiber: 3g; Net carbs: 2g; Protein: 2g

JALAPEÑO POPPERS

SERVES 6 • PREP TIME: 20 MINUTES, PLUS OVERNIGHT SOAKING •
COOK TIME: 20 MINUTES

With these poppers, every day is game day. The "cheese" filling provides a healthy dose of fats and protein for sustained energy. Jalapeños are rich in vitamins A, C, K, and Bs. They also contain potassium and carotene, the latter of which is an antioxidant. It's a touchdown in your mouth and spicy for the win!

Nonstick coconut oil cooking spray

10 jalapeños, halved lengthwise and seeded

1 tablespoon coconut oil

1 cup almonds, soaked overnight

1 teaspoon miso paste

1 teaspoon nutritional yeast

1 teaspoon freshly squeezed lemon juice

1 teaspoon sea salt

2 tablespoons chia seeds

1 tablespoon ground flaxseed

½ cup almond flour

¼ cup coconut flour

¼ cup Raw Keto Ranch (optional, page 43)

1. Preheat the oven to 375°F. Grease a baking sheet with cooking spray and set aside.

2. Place the jalapeños in a mixing bowl and toss with the coconut oil.

3. In a high-powered blender, combine the almonds, miso paste, nutritional yeast, lemon juice, and sea salt, and blend until the mixture is thick, smooth, and creamy. If the mixture is too thin, slowly add water to the blender, drizzling it in until it's well combined. Transfer the mixture to a mixing bowl and place it in the refrigerator for 5 minutes.

4. In a separate mixing bowl, combine the chia seeds, flaxseed, almond flour, and coconut flour. Set aside.

5. Remove the almond mixture from the refrigerator. Using a tablespoon, scoop the mixture into the cavity of a jalapeño, filling it generously.

6. Roll the jalapeño in the flour mixture and place it on the prepared baking sheet. Repeat steps 5 and 6 for the remaining jalapeños.

7. Bake at 375°F for 20 minutes or until the jalapeños are tender and the coating becomes golden and toasty.

8. Serve hot on a platter with the ranch dressing (if using).

SUBSTITUTION TIP: *If you are sensitive to spice, this recipe can easily be made using mini bell peppers instead of jalapeños. The modified version is just as flavorful without the spicy kick.*

Per Serving: Calories: 259; Total fat: 21g; Carbohydrates: 14g; Fiber: 8g; Net carbs: 6g; Protein: 9g

GOURMET "CHEESE" BALLS

SERVES 6 · PREP TIME: 1 HOUR 20 MINUTES, PLUS OVERNIGHT SOAKING

Even dairy cheese lovers will gobble up these savory balls. They're high in fat and protein with an umami goodness that will curb even the unruliest of appetites. You might want to make a double quantity of this recipe because they have a tendency to disappear fast.

1 cup raw hazelnuts, soaked overnight

¼ cup water

2 tablespoons nutritional yeast

1 teaspoon apple cider vinegar

1 teaspoon miso paste

1 teaspoon mustard

½ cup almond flour

1 cup slivered almonds

1 teaspoon dried oregano

1. In a high-powered blender, combine the hazelnuts, water, nutritional yeast, vinegar, miso paste, and mustard, and blend until well combined, thick, and creamy.

2. Transfer the mixture to a medium bowl.

3. Slowly stir in the almond flour until the mixture forms a dough-like consistency. Set aside.

4. In a separate, small bowl, toss the almonds and oregano together and set aside.

5. Using a soup spoon or tablespoon, scoop some mixture into your hand and shape it into a bite-size ball. Place the ball on a baking sheet. Repeat until you have used all the mixture (about 2 dozen balls).

6. One by one, roll the hazelnut balls in the almond and oregano mixture until thoroughly coated, placing each coated ball back on the baking sheet.

7. Place the sheet in the refrigerator for 1 hour to allow the balls to set.

MAKE-AHEAD TIP: *These can be made in advance and stored in an airtight container in the refrigerator for up to 1 week. Freezing is not recommended, as it will alter the texture.*

Per Serving: Calories: 308; Total fat: 27g; Carbohydrates: 11g; Fiber: 6g; Net carbs: 5g; Protein: 10g

OLIVE PÂTÉ

This pâté is fancy enough for company and loaded with heart-healthy fats. Studies have suggested that eating healthy fats before meals can boost metabolic rate and aid in healthy digestion. This pâté is quite elegant when served with some flax crackers or cucumber slices.

1 cup pitted green olives

1 cup pitted black olives

¼ cup cold-pressed olive oil

1 teaspoon freshly ground black pepper

2 thyme sprigs

1. In a food processor, combine all the ingredients and pulse until the mixture is thick and chunky.
2. Transfer the pâté to a small serving bowl and serve with crackers.

COOKING TIP: *This pâté can be easily transformed into a sauce by adding one extra cup of olive oil and a quarter-cup of lemon juice. It tastes amazing over zucchini noodles.*

Per Serving: Calories: 171; Total fat: 17g; Carbohydrates: 4g; Fiber: <1g; Net carbs: 4g; Protein: <1g

AVOCADO "FRIES"

SERVES 6 · PREP TIME: 10 MINUTES · COOK TIME: 15 MINUTES

Avocado lovers unite! The first time each of us had avocado fries we lost our minds over the unique flavor and the simultaneously crunchy and soft textures. Full of omega-9 monounsaturated fat, this dish is not only a looker, it's also good for your heart and skin.

1 or 2 medium semi-firm avocado(s), peeled, pitted, and cut lengthwise into 1-inch-thick sticks

1 cup almond flour

1 tablespoon ground flaxseed

1 teaspoon ground paprika

¼ teaspoon cayenne pepper

1 cup unsweetened hemp milk

1 teaspoon sea salt

1. Preheat the oven to 420°F. Line a baking sheet with parchment paper. If you don't have parchment paper, use aluminum foil or a greased pan.
2. In a mixing bowl, whisk together the almond flour, flaxseed, paprika, and cayenne.
3. Pour the hemp milk into a separate bowl and set aside.
4. Dip the avocado sticks in the hemp milk, then immediately roll them in the dry mixture until well coated. Place the coated avocado sticks on the prepared baking sheet.
5. Bake for 7 minutes on one side, then flip the fries and bake for another 5 minutes until golden brown and crisp.
6. Remove the fries from the oven and sprinkle with the salt.

INGREDIENT TIP: *Dip the fries into any sauce recipe in this book, or sprinkle them with malt vinegar for that classic boathouse flavor. The fries also taste amazing with a bit of lemon juice squeezed over the top.*

Per Serving: Calories: 170; Total fat: 16g; Carbohydrates: 5g; Fiber: 3g; Net carbs: 2g; Protein: 7g

JICAMA NACHOS

SERVES 6 · PREP TIME: 10 MINUTES · COOK TIME: 5 MINUTES

Nachos are the official food group of all major sporting events. We can't explain why, but busting out nachos also busts out the fun. This keto version is very hydrating and much more filling than its high-carb, dairy-based counterpart. The lime, jalapeño, and jicama provide a hit of vitamins, minerals, and antioxidants. This is what winning looks like.

1 lime, halved

½ medium jicama, peeled and thinly sliced

1 cup "Nacho Cheese" Sauce (page 45)

1 small Roma tomato, finely diced

¼ cup finely diced yellow onion

1 jalapeño pepper, seeded and finely diced

¼ cup sliced olives

2 tablespoons coarsely chopped fresh cilantro

1. In a medium bowl, squeeze the lime halves directly over the jicama and set the jicama aside.
2. In a small saucepan, heat the "nacho cheese" until it is warm and a little steam is rising from the surface. If the cheese becomes too thick, stir in a little water to thin it out.
3. Arrange the jicama "nacho chips" on a plate and pour the "nacho cheese" on top.
4. Top with the tomato, onion, and jalapeño.
5. Finish by sprinkling the nachos with the olives and cilantro.

SUBSTITUTION TIP: *If you don't have jicama on hand, you can create the same dish using cucumber or zucchini slices.*

Per Serving: Calories: 79; Total fat: 4g; Carbohydrates: 11g; Fiber: 5gm; Net carbs: 6g; Protein: 3g

SMOKY "HUMMUS" AND VEGGIES

SERVES 6 · PREP TIME: 15 MINUTES ·
COOK TIME: 20 MINUTES, PLUS 20 MINUTES TO CHILL

This dip is a huge crowd pleaser and a perfect option for weekly meal prep. Having it on hand is helpful for those busy weeks when you need something that will quickly satisfy hunger.

Nonstick coconut oil cooking spray

1 cauliflower head, cut into florets

¼ cup tahini

¼ cup cold-pressed olive oil, plus extra for drizzling

Juice of 1 lemon

1 tablespoon ground paprika

1 teaspoon sea salt

¼ cup chopped fresh parsley, for garnish

2 tablespoons pine nuts (optional)

Flax crackers, for serving

Sliced cucumbers, for serving

Celery pieces, for serving

1. Preheat the oven to 400°F and grease a baking sheet with cooking spray.
2. Spread the cauliflower florets out on the prepared baking sheet and bake for 20 minutes.
3. Remove the cauliflower from the oven and allow it to cool for 10 minutes.
4. In a food processor or high-powered blender, combine the cauliflower with the tahini, olive oil, lemon juice, paprika, and salt. Blend on high until a fluffy, creamy texture is achieved. If the mixture seems too thick, slowly add a few tablespoons of water until smooth.
5. Scoop the "hummus" into an airtight container and chill in the refrigerator for about 20 minutes.
6. Transfer the "hummus" to a serving bowl and drizzle with olive oil. Garnish with the parsley and pine nuts (if using).
7. Serve with your favorite flax crackers and sliced cucumbers and celery.

SUBSTITUTION TIP: *For a festive twist on this dip, substitute lemon juice for lime juice and parsley for cilantro. If you like spice, try adding half a jalapeño pepper.*

Per Serving: Calories: 169; Total fat: 15g; Carbohydrates: 9g; Fiber: 4g; Net carbs: 5g; Protein: 4g

FINGER TACOS

SERVES 4 · PREP TIME: 15 MINUTES

Nicole is a big advocate for making healthy snacking fun. This snack involves using nori as a "taco" shell or shovel. Sea vegetables such as nori are a healthy source of iodine, which our body depends on for proper thyroid function. Togarashi is a popular condiment in Japan that contains chile, orange peel, seaweed, ginger, poppy seeds, and sesame seeds. Check the label to make sure it's vegan, as some brands contain shrimp flakes.

2 avocados, peeled and pitted	1 teaspoon ginger powder	10 fresh mint leaves chiffonade
1 lime	1 teaspoon togarashi (optional)	⅓ cup cauliflower rice
1 tablespoon tamari	½ cup kale chiffonade	1 (0.18-ounce) package nori squares or seaweed snack sheets
1 teaspoon sesame oil	½ cup cabbage chiffonade	

1. Put the avocados into a large mixing bowl, and squeeze the lime over them.
2. Roughly mash the avocados with a fork, leaving the mixture fairly chunky.
3. Gently stir in the tamari, sesame oil, ginger powder, and togarashi (if using).
4. Gently fold in the kale, cabbage, mint, and cauliflower rice.
5. Arrange some nori squares on a plate.
6. Use a nori or seaweed sheet to pick up a portion of the avocado mixture and pop it into your mouth.

COOKING TIP: *This dish is easily transformed into an appetizer by omitting the nori and stacking the ingredients on top of flax crackers.*

Per Serving: Calories: 180; Total fat: 15g; Carbohydrates: 13g; Fiber: 8g; Net carbs: 5g; Protein: 4g

FRESH ROSEMARY KETO BREAD

SERVES 6 · PREP TIME: 1 HOUR 45 MINUTES · COOK TIME: 55 MINUTES

Confession: Before diving hard-core into keto, Whitney drove Nicole to a local artisanal bakery for one last hurrah to buy the most expensive loaf of vegan bread they made. Nicole loves bread, but she doesn't always love how it makes her body feel. If you're missing bread, we hear you—and we've got you covered with this recipe. A special note: cane sugar is used in this recipe, but don't worry; it's just to activate the yeast.

1½ cups warm water, divided, plus up to ¼ cup more if needed

1 (¼-ounce) packet active dry yeast

1 teaspoon cane sugar

1 cup coconut flour

3 tablespoons ground psyllium husk

1 rosemary sprig

¾ cup tahini

Sea salt

1. In a small bowl, whisk together ½ cup of warm water with the yeast and sugar. Set aside for 10 minutes to allow the yeast to activate and foam.
2. In a separate small mixing bowl, whisk together the coconut flour, psyllium, and rosemary.
3. In a large mixing bowl, stir together the yeast mixture, tahini, and the remaining 1 cup of warm water.
4. Stir the dry ingredients into the wet ingredients, making sure there are no clumps or dry crumbles. If the dough is crumbly or not well combined, add up to ¼ cup of warm water, 1 tablespoon at a time, until the dough comes together.

5. Line a bread pan with parchment paper and press the dough into the pan. If you don't have parchment paper, use a greased pan. Set the dough to rise in a cool, dark place for 90 minutes. It should rise and expand to double its original size.

6. Preheat the oven to 350°F.

7. Bake the bread for 50 to 55 minutes, or until the crust is firm to the touch.

8. While the bread is still warm, remove it from the pan. Let it cool completely before slicing and serving.

COOKING TIP: *This bread can be transformed into a sweet treat by adding 2 teaspoons of ground cinnamon and ¼ cup of dried blueberries to the dough in step 2.*

Per Serving: Calories: 278; Total fat: 18g; Carbohydrates: 24g; Fiber: 14g; Net carbs: 10g; Protein: 8g

COOKIE FAT BOMBS

SERVES 6 · PREP TIME: 10 MINUTES, PLUS 40 MINUTES TO CHILL

These are the perfect quick pick-me-up that won't let you down. These little balls of magic are high fat, low carb, and utterly delicious, making them the perfect between-meal snack or light dessert. They're so good that even the Cookie Monster would covet them.

1 cup almond butter

½ cup coconut flour

1 teaspoon ground cinnamon

¼ cup cacao nibs or vegan keto chocolate chips

1. Line a baking sheet with parchment paper. If you don't have parchment paper, use aluminum foil or a greased pan.
2. In a mixing bowl, whisk together the almond butter, coconut flour, and cinnamon.
3. Fold in the cacao nibs.
4. Cover the bowl and put it in the freezer for 15 to 20 minutes.
5. Remove the bowl from the freezer and, using a spoon or cookie scoop, scoop out a dollop of mixture and roll it between your palms to form a ball. Repeat to use all the mixture.
6. Place the fat bombs on a baking sheet and put the sheet in the freezer to chill for 20 minutes until firm.

STORAGE TIP: *Store in an airtight container in the refrigerator for 1 to 2 weeks. Keep these bombs on hand to satisfy sudden sugar cravings. They're also great for a pre-workout energy boost.*

Per Serving: Calories: 319; Total fat: 26g; Carbohydrates: 18g; Fiber: 10g; Net carbs: 8g; Protein: 8g

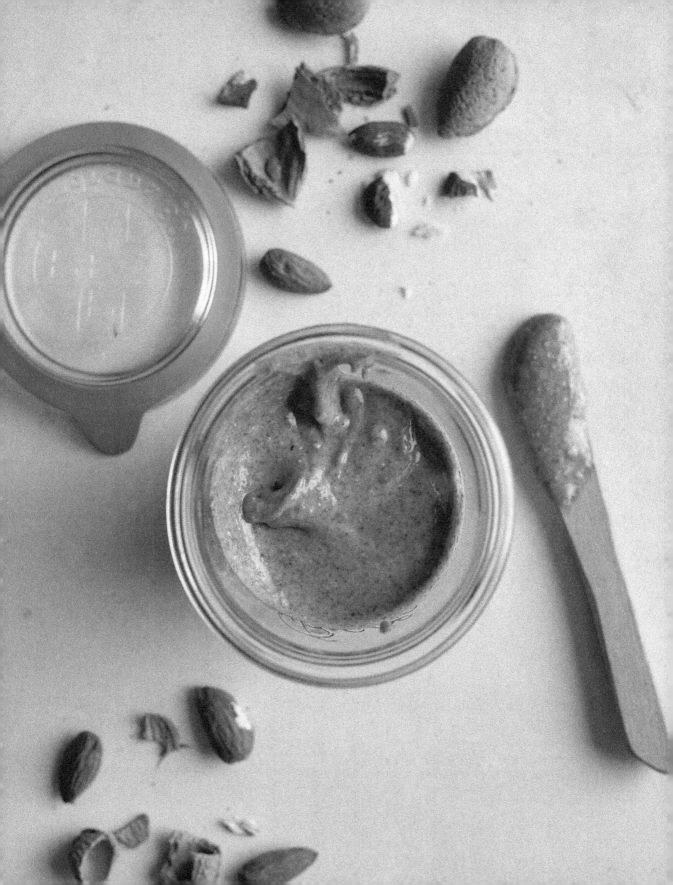

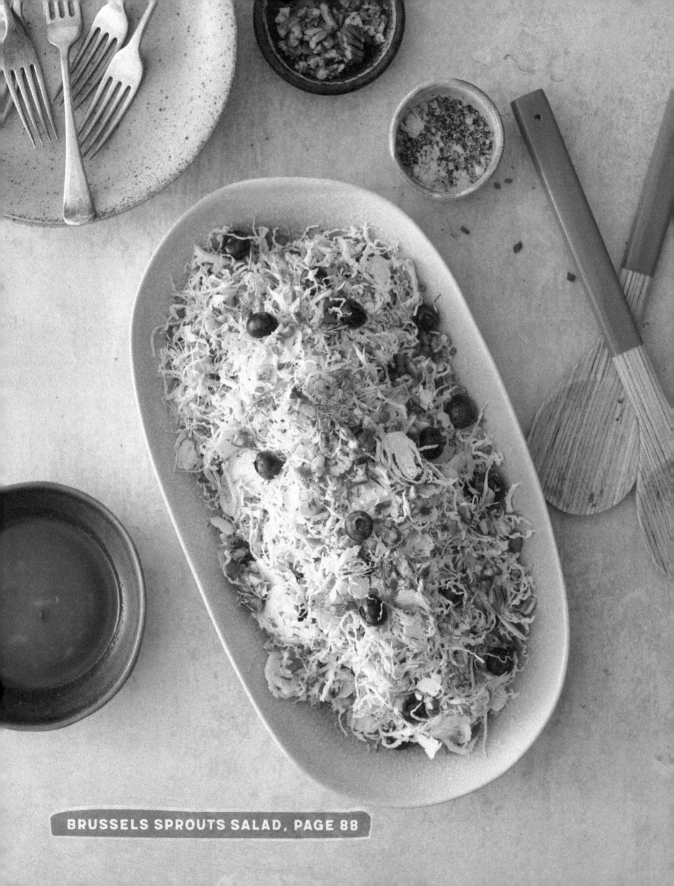

BRUSSELS SPROUTS SALAD, PAGE 88

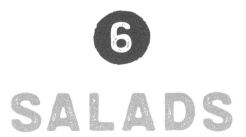

SALADS

There are two kinds of people in this world: those who love salads and eat them frequently, and those who avoid them like the plague. The following recipes were designed for both types. If you adore salads, you're going to relish the mouthwatering combinations of veggies, nuts, seeds, berries, and tantalizing dressings. If you're someone who skips the salad on the menu, we're confident that you'll have a change of heart once you try the following creations.

RAW TABOULI

Traditionally this salad is made with bulgur wheat, but we have swapped it out for cauliflower rice to make this version not only keto but also gluten-free. The parsley in this salad helps alkalize the body by removing heavy metals, and the cauliflower and cucumber are super hydrating.

4 cups cauliflower rice

4 cups chopped fresh parsley

1 cup finely diced tomato

½ cup finely diced yellow onion

2 cups finely diced cucumber

½ cup chopped fresh mint

Juice of 3 lemons

½ cup cold-pressed olive oil

Sea salt

Freshly ground black pepper

1. In a medium bowl, stir together the cauliflower rice, parsley, tomato, onion, cucumber, and mint.

2. Dress with the lemon juice and olive oil, and season with salt and pepper.

3. Place the tabouli in the refrigerator to chill for up to 1 hour to allow the flavors to combine, then serve.

MAKE-AHEAD TIP: *This salad keeps well in an airtight container in the refrigerator. Make it in advance for a quick go-to midweek meal.*

Per Serving: Calories: 317; Total fat: 28g; Carbohydrates: 17g; Fiber: 6g; Net carbs: 11g; Protein: 5g

ASIAN-STYLE CUCUMBER SALAD

SERVES 6 · PREP TIME: 8 MINUTES

Light and easy, this refreshing and hydrating salad is certain to satisfy your hunger. Cucumber is a great vegetable to include in salad, as it is low in carbohydrates and alkalizes the body. Cooking can reduce the alkalizing effect of vegetables, so eating them raw is a nutritious way to enjoy them.

2 large cucumbers, chopped into bite-size cubes

¼ red onion, thinly sliced

½ cup white rice vinegar

1 teaspoon sesame oil

3 or 4 drops liquid stevia

2 tablespoons black sesame seeds

1. Toss the cucumbers and onion together in a large mixing bowl with the vinegar, sesame oil, and stevia.
2. Cover the bowl with plastic wrap or a lid and place the salad in the refrigerator for about 1 hour to marinate.
3. Top the salad with the sesame seeds and serve.

STORAGE TIP: *This salad comes together fast and keeps for up to a week in an airtight container in the refrigerator.*

Per Serving: Calories: 39; Total fat: 2g; Carbohydrates: 4g; Fiber: 1g; Net carbs: 3g; Protein: 1g

BRUSSELS SPROUTS SALAD

SERVES 6 · PREP TIME: 5 MINUTES

Brussels sprouts, those cute little members of the cabbage family, are an incredible source of fiber; one cup gives you 4 grams. They also provide a hit of iron and a generous dose of vitamins A and C. All the more reason to make this salad, which can be tossed together in a jiffy for some fall flavor.

6 cups shredded Brussels sprouts

1 cup chopped pecans

⅓ cup chopped fresh chives

3 tablespoons chopped fresh dill

½ cup cold-pressed olive oil

Juice of 1 lemon

1 teaspoon sea salt

1 teaspoon freshly ground black pepper

⅓ cup fresh blueberries

1. Toss the Brussels sprouts with the pecans, chives, and dill.
2. In a small bowl or jar, whisk together the olive oil, lemon juice, salt. and pepper.
3. Toss the salad with the dressing, top with the blueberries, and serve.

SUBSTITUTION TIP: *For a warm version of this salad, leave the blueberries out. Prepare the ingredients and place them on a greased baking sheet. Broil under medium heat for a few minutes, just enough to toast the edges of the sprouts and warm the salad.*

Per Serving: Calories: 349; Total fat: 32g; Carbohydrates: 13g; Fiber: 5g; Net carbs: 8g; Protein: 2g

BROCCOLI & RASPBERRY "BACON" SALAD

SERVES 6 • PREP TIME: 5 MINUTES

This salad is on heavy rotation in Nicole's home. It's her vegan keto answer to the classic southern broccoli salad. You know—the one with bacon. She substitutes freeze-dried raspberries and paprika to get bacon's signature smoky flavor. Broccoli keeps your bones strong, is thought to help prevent cancer, and can boost your immune system.

4 tablespoons tahini

Juice of 2 lemons

1 tablespoon apple cider vinegar

1 tablespoon paprika

1 teaspoon cayenne pepper (optional)

Sea salt

Freshly ground black pepper

1 pound broccoli florets

¼ red onion, finely chopped

⅓ cup freeze-dried raspberries, crushed

1. In a medium mixing bowl, whisk together the tahini, lemon juice, vinegar, paprika, and cayenne, and season with salt and pepper.

2. In a large bowl, toss the broccoli with the onion.

3. Top the vegetables with the tahini mixture and toss vigorously to coat.

4. Sprinkle the raspberries on top and toss again.

5. Allow to marinate in the refrigerator for at least 1 hour, and overnight for the best result.

COOKING TIP: *If you are sensitive to the bloating typically associated with cruciferous vegetables, prepare this salad a day in advance. The acidity from the apple cider vinegar will start to break down the broccoli, which "cooks" it the same way citrus "cooks" the fish in ceviche.*

Per Serving: Calories: 99; Total fat: 6g; Carbohydrates: 9g; Fiber: 3g; Net carbs: 6g; Protein: 3g

CITRUS ARUGULA SALAD

SERVES 4 · PREP TIME: 5 MINUTES

This elegant salad contains the low-carb fruit grapefruit. It provides a walloping 64 percent of the daily requirement of immune system-boosting vitamin C. It also contains flavonoids to help protect you against cancer, as does arugula, which also promotes bone growth through its calcium content.

1 pound arugula, washed

⅓ cup cold-pressed olive oil

Juice of 1 lemon

Sea salt

Freshly ground black pepper

1 avocado, cubed

½ grapefruit, peeled and sliced

¼ cup pine nuts

1. Dress the arugula lightly with the olive oil and lemon juice, and season with salt and pepper.
2. Add the avocado and grapefruit to the dressed arugula.
3. Top with the pine nuts and serve.

INGREDIENT TIP: *This salad is a good option for anyone working to heal high blood pressure. Grapefruit is low in carbohydrates, making it a perfect keto option, and rich in antioxidants to support healthy heart function.*

Per Serving: Calories: 328; Total fat: 31g; Carbohydrates: 12g; Fiber: 5g; Net carbs: 7g; Protein: 5g

KALE CAESAR

The first time Nicole had a Caesar salad, she was a little girl eating at a high-end hotel restaurant to celebrate turning double digits. She recalls her fascination while watching the side-table construction of the salad and its elaborate presentation. It was as if she were seeing a theatrical production unfold before her eyes. Enjoy her upgraded keto take on this iconic classic.

1 bunch kale, stems removed, leaves cut into ribbons

3 tablespoons cold-pressed olive oil

Juice of 1 lemon

½ cup Vegan "Sour Cream" (page 46)

3 tablespoons capers

3 tablespoons shredded seaweed

1 teaspoon Old Bay seasoning

1 teaspoon freshly ground black pepper

Sea salt

1 ripe avocado, peeled, pitted, and sliced

3 tablespoons pepitas (pumpkin seeds)

1 teaspoon nutritional yeast

1. Put the kale in a large mixing bowl and drizzle with the olive oil.
2. Massage the oil into the kale, rubbing it between your hands until the leaves become tender and shiny.
3. Pour the lemon juice over the massaged kale and set aside.
4. In a small mixing bowl, whisk together the "sour cream," capers, seaweed, Old Bay seasoning, and pepper, and season with salt to create the dressing.
5. Toss the massaged kale in the dressing and divide among small serving bowls.
6. Top each bowl with the avocado, pepitas, and nutritional yeast.

MAKE-AHEAD TIP: *Kale is a strong and wilt-resistant green. This is the perfect salad to make ahead on your weekly meal-prep day. It will stay fresh for up to 4 days.*

Per Serving: Calories: 338; Total fat: 28g; Carbohydrates: 23g; Fiber: 9g; Net carbs: 14g; Protein: 10g

BIG GREEK SPINACH SALAD

SERVES 4 · PREP TIME: 5 MINUTES

In Greece this traditional salad is called horiatiki, which translates to "village salad." It's light, and yet the olives pack in nutritional density to make this salad refreshing, hydrating, and completely satisfying. We have omitted the traditional feta to make our version vegan, but you won't miss it. If you prefer to add in cheese, keep an eye out for a vegan feta in the refrigerated section of markets or order it online. Opa!

½ cup cold-pressed olive oil

Juice of 1 lemon

1 tablespoon dried mint

1 tablespoon dried oregano

Sea salt

Freshly ground black pepper

1 cup cubed, drained, firm sprouted tofu

1 medium cucumber, sliced

½ cup cherry tomatoes, halved

½ green bell pepper, sliced

¼ small red onion, thinly sliced

¼ cup coarsely chopped fresh mint

5 cups fresh spinach, chopped

1 head romaine lettuce, chopped

⅓ cup sliced olives

¼ cup pine nuts

1. In a medium mixing bowl, whisk together the olive oil, lemon juice, mint, and oregano, and season with salt and pepper.

2. Toss the tofu in the dressing and set aside to marinate.

3. In a separate medium bowl, toss together the cucumber, tomatoes, bell pepper, onion, and mint.

4. Add the spinach, lettuce, and olives.

5. Add the dressed tofu. Toss salad again.

6. Serve the salad in small bowls, garnished with the olives and pine nuts.

MAKE-AHEAD TIP: *To batch out this salad for meal prep, leave the spinach out until you are ready to eat the salad. When the time comes, dump the other components over the spinach, toss, and serve. This will allow you to prepare the salad in advance but also ensure the spinach will not be wilted.*

Per Serving: Calories: 406; Total fat: 38g; Carbohydrates: 13g; Fiber: 6g; Net carbs: 7g; Protein: 10g

FIESTA SALAD

They say we eat first with our eyes, and this salad is a beautiful feast to look at. While it packs a killer color punch, it's also rich in vitamin C to keep you healthy and dancing. The high seed content adds a nutritional and satisfying crunch.

1 head romaine lettuce, chopped

⅓ cup diced red bell pepper

⅓ cup diced yellow bell pepper

⅓ cup diced orange bell pepper

¼ cup chopped fresh cilantro

⅓ cup Ginger-Lime Dressing (page 48)

Sea salt

Freshly ground black pepper

1 teaspoon ground cumin

3 tablespoons pepitas

1 avocado, peeled, pitted, and cubed

4 or 5 flax crackers, broken into pieces

1. In a medium bowl, combine the romaine, bell peppers, and cilantro.
2. Toss the salad with the dressing, and season with salt, pepper, and the cumin.
3. Divide among individual serving bowls and top each bowl with the avocado, pepitas, and flax cracker pieces.

SUBSTITUTION TIP: *If you are feeling low in iron, you can substitute out the romaine. Kale is an excellent, iron-packed alternative green, making it an especially good choice for athletes.*

Per Serving: Calories: 308; Total fat: 28g; Carbohydrates: 11g; Fiber: 6g; Net carbs: 5g; Protein: 6g

KALE, AVOCADO & TAHINI SALAD

SERVES 4 · PREP TIME: 5 MINUTES

If you were stranded on an island and could only eat one thing for the rest of your life, what would it be? This is Nicole's choice, hands down. Not only does it satisfy on so many fronts—hello, creamy and crunchy—it's also astoundingly detoxifying. Choose this salad when you are feeling a little rundown and in need of a boost.

1 bunch kale, stems removed, leaves cut into ribbons

¼ cup cold-pressed olive oil

4 to 5 tablespoons Tahini Goddess dressing (page 49)

1 avocado, peeled, pitted, and sliced

¼ cup slivered almonds

3 tablespoons chia seeds

1. In a large mixing bowl, coat the kale with the olive oil. Massage the leaves with your hands to tenderize them and remove bitterness.

2. Toss the massaged kale with the dressing.

3. Divide the salad among 4 bowls and top each bowl with the avocado, almonds, and chia seeds.

MAKE-AHEAD TIP: *This salad does perfectly as a make-ahead item, so double the recipe and store half in an airtight container in the refrigerator. The kale will keep its texture for up to 3 days.*

Per Serving: Calories: 370; Total fat: 30g; Carbohydrates: 22g; Fiber: 12g; Net carbs: 10g; Protein: 9g

VEGAN NIÇOISE SALAD

SERVES 4 · PREP TIME: 10 MINUTES

For this upgraded version of the French classic, we have omitted the eggs and fish to make it vegan. As you crunch away, allow yourself to be transported to a cottage nook. Look out the window and take in the French countryside as the breeze kisses your face. Magnifique!

15 to 20 fresh green beans

3 small heads butter lettuce, coarsely chopped

⅓ cup Herb Garden Dressing (page 47)

1 small cucumber, chopped

1 small tomato, chopped

¼ cup olives

5 radishes, chopped

1. Pour water into a medium bowl and add a generous amount of ice. Set aside.
2. In a medium saucepan over high heat, bring plenty of water to a boil.
3. Toss the green beans into the pot and blanch them for 3 minutes.
4. Remove the green beans from the water and immediately submerge them in the ice-water bath to preserve their color and crunch.
5. Toss the butter lettuce with the dressing and divide among 4 bowls. Top each bowl with the green beans, cucumber, tomato, olives, and radishes.

COOKING TIP: *To save time, instead of boiling the green beans, place them in a bowl and cover them with a wet towel. Microwave for 60 seconds and you are good to go.*

Per Serving: Calories: 153; Total fat: 13g; Carbohydrates: 9g; Fiber: 3g; Net carbs: 6g; Protein: 3g

KETO COBB SALAD

SERVES 4 · PREP TIME: 5 MINUTES

In 1937, Amelia Earhart disappeared, Morgan Freeman was born, and the cousin of baseball great Ty Cobb created this American classic at the legendary Brown Derby restaurant in Los Angeles. This hodgepodge of leftover ingredients is also salad's most photogenic family member. Here we present a reimagining of a familiar staple that is loaded with nutritional benefits.

1 (14-ounce) block firm tofu

3 tablespoons tahini

3 tablespoons nutritional yeast

1 teaspoon kala namak salt

1 teaspoon turmeric powder

8 cups mixed greens

1 medium tomato, chopped

1 avocado, peeled, pitted, and chopped

⅓ cup chopped yellow onion

1 small cucumber, chopped

⅓ cup chopped red bell pepper

⅓ cup Coconut "Bacon" (see page 98)

3 tablespoons hemp seeds

⅓ cup Raw Keto Ranch (page 43)

1. Drain the tofu, place it on a cutting board or plate, and press to remove as much water as possible.

2. Crumble the tofu into a medium mixing bowl and toss it with the tahini, nutritional yeast, kala namak salt, and turmeric to create "egg" crumbles.

3. On 4 serving plates, arrange the greens, tomato, avocado, onion, cucumber, bell pepper, "egg" crumbles, coconut "bacon," and hemp seeds.

4. Drizzle with the dressing and serve.

LEFTOVERS TIP: *If you have extra "egg" crumbles, store them in the refrigerator. The "egg" mixture makes a great breakfast when pan-fried and served with avocado and flaxseed crackers.*

Per Serving: Calories: 406; Total fat: 28g; Carbohydrates: 22g; Fiber: 11g; Net carbs: 11g; Protein: 22g

JAPANESE HIBACHI HOUSE SALAD

SERVES 6 · PREP TIME: 5 MINUTES

Thanks to the carrots in the dressing for this salad, you'll get a big boost of vitamin A. This root vegetable is also rich in beta carotene and amino acids. The ginger will combat inflammation. Sesame seeds are a good source of several nutrients, such as zinc, iron, and selenium, and vitamins B6 and E. Keep sesame seeds refrigerated or frozen to avoid them turning rancid, which can happen due to their high oil content.

1-inch knob fresh ginger, peeled and chopped

½ medium carrot

½ celery stalk

Juice of 2 limes

¼ cup liquid aminos

1 teaspoon sesame oil

3 drops liquid stevia

2 heads romaine lettuce, chopped

1 small tomato, diced

½ cup sliced mushrooms

⅓ cup shredded carrots

⅓ cup diced red onion

2 tablespoons sesame seeds

1. In a high-powered blender, combine the ginger, carrot, celery, lime juice, aminos, sesame oil, and liquid stevia to create the dressing.
2. Divide the lettuce among 6 bowls and top each bowl with a generous portion of dressing. Garnish with the tomato, mushrooms, shredded carrots, onion, and sesame seeds.

LEFTOVERS TIP: *Extra dressing can be stored in the refrigerator for up to 1 week. Keep it handy to dress up other last-minute meals or as a dip for raw vegetables.*

Per Serving: Calories: 65; Total fat: 3g; Carbohydrates: 8g; Fiber: 4g; Net carbs: 4g; Protein: 4g

RANCH WEDGE SALAD WITH COCONUT "BACON"

SERVES 6 · PREP TIME: 15 MINUTES · COOK TIME: 25 MINUTES

Something about having to get out a fork and knife to cut into this salad makes it feel like a really substantial meal. Traditionally this salad is served with bacon and blue cheese, but we swapped those items out to make this wedge completely vegan and keto-friendly. The coconut "bacon" is a terrific stand-in and, dare we say it, even better than the original.

FOR THE COCONUT "BACON"

4 tablespoons liquid smoke

½ cup tamari

½ cup cold-pressed olive oil

½ cup monk fruit sweetener

1 tablespoon ground paprika

4 cups dried coconut flakes

FOR THE SALAD

1 head iceberg lettuce, cut into 6 wedges

½ cup Raw Keto Ranch (page 43)

1 small tomato, chopped

¼ cup chopped fresh chives

Sea salt

Freshly ground black pepper

TO MAKE THE COCONUT "BACON"

1. Preheat the oven to 375°F, line a baking sheet with a silicone mat or parchment paper, and spray with cooking spray. If you don't have parchment paper, use aluminum foil or a greased pan.
2. In a large skillet over medium heat, whisk together the liquid smoke, tamari, olive oil, monk fruit sweetener, and paprika. Stir the mixture occasionally to melt the sweetener.

3. Once the sweetener is dissolved, toss in the coconut flakes and cook for 5 minutes, allowing the liquid to evaporate.

4. Remove the coconut flakes from the skillet and transfer to the prepared baking sheet, spreading the coconut out evenly.

5. Bake for 20 minutes or until the edges become toasted, then remove the sheet from the oven and set aside to cool.

TO MAKE THE SALAD

Top the lettuce wedges with the dressing and garnish with the tomato, chives, and coconut "bacon." Season with salt and pepper and serve.

MAKE-AHEAD TIP: *The coconut "bacon" from this dish can be made in advance and stored in a sealed container as a pantry item. Sprinkle coconut "bacon" on anything to give it some extra pizzazz.*

Per Serving: Calories: 500; Total fat: 48g; Carbohydrates: 18g; Fiber: 8g; Net carbs: 10g; Protein: 8g

THAI TUM YUM SOUP, PAGE 113

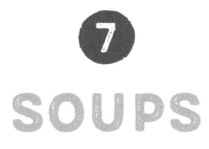

SOUPS

During the cold seasons, soup warms us up from the inside out. When it's hot outside, there's nothing like a refreshing cup of chilled soup. And don't forget the tradition of eating chili while watching a good sports game. Soups are great year-round, and you don't have to skip them on the vegan keto diet. You can slurp up most of the classic flavors you've always loved.

GAZPACHO

Gazpacho originally hails from the Andalusian region in northern Spain. Chilled soups are perfect for hot days or when you prefer to sip your vegetables. This gazpacho is loaded with vitamin C and is wonderfully refreshing and hydrating.

3 medium heirloom tomatoes, coarsely chopped

2 garlic cloves, diced

2 medium cucumbers, peeled and coarsely chopped

1 shallot, coarsely chopped

½ red bell pepper, coarsely chopped

½ cup coarsely chopped fresh cilantro, plus more for garnish

¼ cup cold-pressed olive oil

1 teaspoon apple cider vinegar

½ jalapeño pepper, coarsely chopped (optional)

Freshly ground black pepper

3 cups water, chilled

1. Combine the tomatoes, garlic, cucumbers, shallot, bell pepper, cilantro, olive oil, vinegar, and jalapeño (if using), in a high-powered blender, and blend until smooth. Season with black pepper.
2. Slowly add the water while blending, until your desired consistency is reached. The soup should be slightly thick and easy to sip.
3. Chill the gazpacho in the refrigerator for 1 hour.
4. Serve in wine goblets for a beautiful presentation, garnished with cracked black pepper and a sprinkling of chopped cilantro.

COOKING TIP: *To chill soup faster, replace the chilled water with ice cubes. Allow them to dissolve into the soup until it reaches the desired temperature. Add more water if needed.*

Per Serving: Calories: 85; Total fat: 7g; Carbohydrates: 5g; Fiber: 1g; Net carbs: 4g; Protein: 1g

TOMATO BISQUE

SERVES 8 · PREP TIME: 10 MINUTES · COOK TIME: 40 MINUTES

When Nicole was little and her mom worked the graveyard shift, this was her dad's go-to meal. He spoiled the kids with carpet picnics of grilled cheese sandwiches and tomato soup. This grown-up version always brings back sweet memories to Nicole, and we hope it will become a new tradition for you.

Nonstick coconut oil cooking spray

1 pound heirloom cherry tomatoes, coarsely chopped

1 yellow onion, coarsely chopped

2 garlic cloves, coarsely chopped

¼ cup cold-pressed olive oil, plus more for drizzling

2 thyme sprigs

Sea salt

Freshly ground black pepper

1 lemon, halved

1 cup coconut cream

⅓ cup chopped fresh basil, for garnish

1. Preheat the oven to 400°F. Grease a baking dish with cooking spray and set aside.

2. Combine the tomatoes, onion, and garlic in the baking dish. Drizzle with the olive oil and toss in the thyme. Season with salt and pepper. Top with the lemon halves and roast for 20 minutes or until the tomatoes start to blister.

3. Remove from the oven and transfer the mixture to a large saucepan over low heat.

4. Stir in the coconut cream and bring the soup to a simmer. Cook for 20 minutes to allow the flavors to meld together.

5. Remove and discard the lemon halves.

6. Turn off the heat and blend the soup with an immersion blender until it is silky smooth (adding warm water if necessary to reach desired texture).

7. Finish with cracked black pepper, olive oil drizzle, the basil, and additional salt, if desired.

SUBSTITUTION TIP: *If you want to make this soup outside of tomato season, the heirloom tomatoes can be swapped out for any varietal of cherry tomatoes. Avoid using Roma or beefsteak tomatoes as they are typically less sweet and won't yield the same flavor.*

Per Serving: Calories: 142; Total fat: 14g; Carbohydrates: 7g; Fiber: 2g; Net carbs: 5g; Protein: 1g

SPRING PEA SOUP

SERVES 8 · PREP TIME: 5 MINUTES · COOK TIME: 15 MINUTES

Peas are generally not included in the keto diet. However, we made them work in this low-carb recipe as a special treat. They are loaded with protein and help improve digestion while lowering inflammation in the body. Traditional split pea soup is made with ham and dried peas. Our version is lighter, and the use of fresh peas loads the dish with protein, iron, and vitamin B.

3 tablespoons coconut oil

2 shallots, chopped

2 thyme sprigs

Sea salt

Freshly ground black pepper

4 cups fresh peas (frozen, if out of season)

8 cups vegetable broth

¼ cup chopped fresh mint

Juice of 1 lemon

Fresh pea shoots, for garnish

1. Heat the coconut oil in a large stockpot over medium heat.
2. Toss in the shallots and the thyme. Season with salt and pepper.
3. Sauté until the shallots becomes tender, about 3 minutes.
4. Add the peas to the pan; stir to coat them with the oil, and allow them to toast.
5. Add the vegetable broth and bring to a simmer.
6. Remove the pot from the heat and stir in the mint and lemon juice.
7. Using an immersion blender, blend the soup until silky smooth.
8. Garnish with fresh pea shoots and serve hot.

COOKING TIP: *This recipe is simple and quick to make. For a brighter presentation and color, add the peas after you have turned off the heat and before using the immersion blender. This will yield a bright green soup.*

Per Serving: Calories: 124; Total fat: 5g; Carbohydrates: 15g; Fiber: 5g; Net carbs: 10g; Protein: 4g

CREAMY LEEK SOUP

SERVES 8 · PREP TIME: 10 MINUTES · COOK TIME: 30 MINUTES

This soup packs a lot of comfort, thanks in part to the fat in the coconut cream. It is perfect for chilly fall nights or when your officemate decides to blast the air conditioning and turn your work environment into a polar den. And bonus: The onion, leek, herbs, and lemon juice will help ward off a cold.

¼ cup cold-pressed olive oil

1 yellow onion, coarsely chopped

Sea salt

3 cups coarsely chopped cauliflower

1 leek, white and pale green parts only, coarsely chopped

8 cups vegetable broth

1 cup coconut cream

2 rosemary sprigs

2 thyme sprigs

1 bay leaf

Juice of 1 lemon

Freshly ground black pepper

1. In a large stockpot over medium heat, warm the olive oil and add the onion. Season with salt. Sauté until the onion becomes translucent, about 3 minutes.

2. Add the cauliflower and leek and stir for 5 minutes.

3. Add the vegetable broth, coconut cream, rosemary, thyme, and bay leaf, and bring to a low simmer.

4. Simmer for 20 minutes until the vegetables are extremely tender, then remove the pot from the heat and add the lemon juice.

5. Fish out the rosemary and thyme sprigs and the bay leaf, then, using an immersion blender, blend the soup until silky smooth, adding a little water if needed.

6. Garnish with fresh cracked black pepper. Serve hot.

USE IT AGAIN TIP: *Turn any additional cauliflower into keto "rice." Place the chopped cauliflower in a high-powered blender or food processor and pulse until it is in rice-like pieces. Store in a glass container in the refrigerator and use it to make veggie bowls.*

Per Serving: Calories: 158; Total fat: 13g; Carbohydrates: 9g; Fiber: 3g; Net carbs: 6g; Protein: 1g

BUTTERNUT SQUASH SOUP WITH TURMERIC & GINGER

SERVES 8 · PREP TIME: 5 MINUTES · COOK TIME: 35 MINUTES

Nothing says cozy comfort more than an epic butternut squash soup. We added lemongrass for extra layers of flavor. The ginger and turmeric are anti-inflammatory and add a warmth to this lovely and colorful soup.

- 1 small butternut squash
- 3 tablespoons coconut oil
- 3 shallots, coarsely chopped
- 1-inch knob fresh ginger, peeled and coarsely chopped
- 1-inch knob fresh turmeric root, peeled and coarsely chopped
- 1 fresh lemongrass stalk, coarsely chopped
- ½ cup dry Marsala wine (optional)
- 8 cups miso broth
- 1 cup coconut cream
- Cold-pressed olive oil, for drizzling
- Handful toasted pumpkin seeds, for garnish (optional)

1. Preheat the oven to 365°F.
2. Puncture the squash skin with a fork several times to create air vents. Put the entire squash into a baking dish and bake for 30 minutes or until it is extremely tender.
3. While the squash is baking, heat the oil in a large stockpot over medium heat. Add the shallots, ginger, turmeric, and lemongrass to the pan and sauté until the spices become fragrant and the shallots are tender.
4. Deglaze the pot by pouring in the Marsala wine (if using), and stirring, scraping the bottom of the pot to loosen any stuck bits. Once the alcohol starts to reduce, add the miso broth and turn the heat to low.

5. Remove the squash from oven and poke it with a fork to check for tenderness. Carefully cut the squash in half lengthwise, allowing any liquid to drain out.

6. Once the squash is cool enough to handle, scoop out the seeds. With a paring knife, remove the skin. Roughly chop the squash and add it to the stockpot.

7. Pour the coconut cream into the pot, bring to a simmer, and remove from the heat.

8. Using an immersion blender, blend the soup thoroughly until smooth and velvety. Drizzle with olive oil, and top with toasted pumpkin seeds, if desired. Serve warm.

INGREDIENT TIP: *To make this a cold-busting soup, double the ginger, squeeze in fresh lemon juice, and add a couple of handfuls of raw spinach.*

Per Serving: Calories: 149; Total fat: 13g; Carbohydrates: 10g; Fiber: 1g; Net carbs: 9g; Protein: 2g

MISO MAGIC

SERVES 8 • PREP TIME: 5 MINUTES • COOK TIME: 10 MINUTES

This is a great soup for those times when you feel the need to replenish your body, such as recovery from physical trauma, intense workouts, or general depletion. It settles the stomach while re-mineralizing the body.

8 cups water

6 to 7 tablespoons miso paste

3 sheets dried seaweed

2 cups thinly sliced shiitake mushrooms

1 cup drained and cubed sprouted tofu

1 cup chopped scallions

1 teaspoon sesame oil

1. In a large stockpot over medium heat, add the miso paste and seaweed to the water and bring to a low boil.
2. Toss in the mushrooms, tofu, scallions, and sesame oil.
3. Allow to simmer for about 5 minutes and serve.

COOKING TIP: *If you are feeling worn down and in need of an iron boost, simply add 2 cups of torn spinach to your hot soup when you add the tofu.*

Per Serving: Calories: 80; Total fat: 2g; Carbohydrates: 12g; Fiber: 2g; Net carbs: 10g; Protein: 4g

AVOCADO-LIME SOUP

SERVES 8 · PREP TIME: 5 MINUTES · COOK TIME: 20 MINUTES

This soup has a festive flair, making it the perfect lunchtime or dinnertime pick-me-up. Whether you are building an empire or planning your next epic nap, you need those omegas, and this soup is chock-full of them.

2 tablespoons cold-pressed olive oil

½ yellow onion, chopped

1 teaspoon ground cumin

1 teaspoon ground coriander

1 teaspoon chili powder

¼ cup hemp hearts

1 medium tomato, chopped

1 cup chopped cabbage (set some aside for garnish)

½ cup chopped fresh cilantro

½ cup chopped celery

½ jalapeño pepper, chopped

8 cups vegetable broth

Juice of 2 limes

1 avocado, peeled, pitted, and cut into cubes

3 flax crackers

1. Heat the olive oil in a large stockpot over medium heat and add the onion, cumin, coriander, and chili powder. Sauté, stirring occasionally, until the onion becomes tender, about 5 minutes.
2. Add the hemp hearts, tomato, cabbage, cilantro, celery, and jalapeño to the pot. Stir to coat the spices and allow to cook for 4 minutes.
3. Pour the broth into the pot and simmer on low for 20 minutes.
4. Remove the pot from the heat and stir in the lime juice.
5. Divide the avocado equally among 4 serving bowls.
6. Pour the soup over the avocado in the bowls and garnish with additional cabbage and cilantro.
7. Break the flax crackers over the top of the soup to create a "tortilla soup" vibe.

INGREDIENT TIP: *When shopping for the perfect avocado, it's important to test for ripeness. Hold the fruit in your hand and give it a gentle squeeze. If the avocado gives to your touch, it's ready to be eaten. If it's too firm, store it in a brown paper bag on the countertop for a day or so until the avocado has ripened.*

Per Serving: Calories: 130; Total fat: 9g; Carbohydrates: 9g; Fiber: 4g; Net carbs: 5g; Protein: 3g

TUSCAN KALE SOUP

Kale is one of the world's best sources of vitamin K, and is also rich in iron and other antioxidants to help prevent aging and disease. We like to sneak kale into our meals whenever we get the chance.

¼ cup cold-pressed olive oil

½ cup finely diced yellow onion

2 garlic cloves, chopped

2 tablespoons dried oregano

8 cups vegetable broth

¼ cup hemp hearts

3 cups lacinato kale, stems removed, and leaves cut into thin ribbons

1 cup chopped fresh parsley, plus a few sprigs for garnish

½ cup diced rutabaga

⅓ cup diced sun-dried tomatoes

⅓ cup diced carrot

Juice of 1 lemon

Sea salt

1. In a large stockpot over medium heat, heat the olive oil.
2. Add the onion, garlic, and oregano and cook, stirring frequently to prevent sticking, until the onion is tender and the garlic is fragrant, about 5 minutes.
3. Pour the broth into the pot and turn the heat to low.
4. After the broth has been simmering for about 5 minutes, toss in the hemp hearts and simmer for another 15 minutes.
5. Add the kale, parsley, rutabaga, sun-dried tomatoes, and carrot and simmer for another 5 minutes until the carrots are tender.
6. Remove the pot from the heat and squeeze in the lemon juice, then throw in the entire lemon peel to allow the oils from the skin to get into the broth. Season with salt.
7. Garnish the soup with parsley sprigs and serve hot.

SUBSTITUTION TIP: *If you're not a big fan of kale, swap it out for collard greens or spinach. Both options will provide vitamin C and iron.*

Per Serving: Calories: 139; Total fat: 9g; Carbohydrates: 11g; Fiber: 3g; Net carbs: 8g; Protein: 3g

ITALIAN WEDDING SOUP

SERVES 8 · PREP TIME: 10 MINUTES · COOK TIME: 15 MINUTES

We're lovers of fresh herbs and microgreens. They pack a huge punch of fresh flavor and are incredibly beneficial to your health. And since there aren't any meatballs in this vegan keto version, we've upped the iron by including tons of parsley and spinach.

1 tablespoon coconut oil

½ cup coarsely chopped yellow onion

1 teaspoon freshly ground black pepper

1 teaspoon dried oregano

1 bay leaf

⅓ cup coarsely chopped daikon radish

⅓ cup cauliflower rice

½ cup coarsely chopped celery

8 cups vegetable broth

3 cups coarsely chopped fresh Italian parsley

3 cups coarsely chopped spinach

Juice of 1 lemon

1. Warm the coconut oil in a large soup pot over medium heat.
2. Add the onion, pepper, oregano, and bay leaf to the pot and sauté until the onion is translucent, about 3 minutes.
3. Add the daikon, cauliflower rice, and celery to the pot and cook, stirring occasionally, for 5 minutes.
4. Pour the vegetable broth over the sautéed vegetables and bring to a simmer.
5. Remove the pot from the heat and stir in the parsley, spinach, and lemon juice. Serve hot.

MAKE-AHEAD TIP: *Make a double batch and store half in the freezer for quick meals. When you're ready to enjoy it, place it in a pot and warm it up on the stove.*

Per Serving: Calories: 51; Total fat: 2g; Carbohydrates: 7g; Fiber: 3g; Net carbs: 4g; Protein: 1g

FRENCH ONION SOUP

SERVES 8 · PREP TIME: 10 MINUTES · COOK TIME: 1 HOUR

Traditional French onion soup is made with beef broth, butter, and three types of cheese, plus crusty French bread to soak up every last drop. This vegan version is equally decadent, but a lot more nutritious. It's a great choice to make, and serve if you want to impress dinner guests. With the soup casually simmering in the background, your kitchen will smell heavenly.

¼ cup cold-pressed olive oil

3 garlic cloves, chopped

3 thyme sprigs

2 red onions, peeled and thinly sliced

1 yellow onion, peeled and thinly sliced

1 cup dry Marsala wine

8 cups vegetable broth

Salt (optional)

1. Heat the oil in a large stockpot over low heat.
2. Add the garlic and thyme and cook until the garlic becomes fragrant, about 3 minutes.
3. Stir in the red and yellow onions, and caramelize the mixture slowly on low heat, stirring occasionally to prevent them from burning.
4. Once the onions have taken on a dark brown color, add the Marsala wine, stirring and scraping the bottom of the pan to deglaze it.
5. Add the vegetable broth and simmer on low for 60 minutes; this will give the soup a wonderfully rich taste. Add extra broth or water if needed. Note: the liquid in the pot will reduce.
6. Remove the pot from the heat and taste, adding salt if desired.
7. Finish with a drizzle of olive oil and serve hot.

COOKING TIP: *To add extra decadence to this soup, top with a vegan mozzarella (our favorite brand is Miyoko's). Put soup in an oven-safe dish and broil under high heat in the oven until the cheese is toasted.*

Per Serving: Calories: 113; Total fat: 8g; Carbohydrates: 8g; Fiber: 2g; Net carbs: 6g; Protein: 4g

THAI TUM YUM SOUP

In Nicole's hometown there was a quaint Thai restaurant that she and her sister went to regularly once they were old enough to drive. The food instilled in them a taste for food from far-off lands. This recipe for Tom Yum Soup, or as we like to call it—Tum Yum Soup—is the vegan keto version of one of our favorite dishes.

8 cups vegetable broth

1-inch knob fresh ginger, peeled and diced

2 garlic cloves, diced

1 teaspoon galangal

2 kefir lime leaves

1 cup coconut cream

1 cup sliced mushrooms

1 Roma tomato, coarsely chopped

½ yellow onion, coarsely chopped

1 cup coarsely chopped broccoli

1 cup coarsely chopped cauliflower

1 cup chopped fresh cilantro, for garnish

1 lime, cut into wedges, for garnish

1. In a large stockpot over medium heat, bring the broth to a simmer with the ginger, garlic, galangal, and lime leaves.

2. Pour in the coconut cream, followed by the mushrooms, tomato, onion, broccoli, and cauliflower. Simmer until tender.

3. Remove the pot from the heat and serve the soup garnished with the cilantro and a lime slice.

SUBSTITUTION TIP: *For a lighter version of this soup, omit the coconut cream. A good substitute is half an avocado to ensure you're getting plenty of healthy fat.*

Per Serving: Calories: 97; Total fat: 7g; Carbohydrates: 9g; Fiber: 3g; Net carbs: 6g; Protein: 1g

VEGAN PHO

Pho originated in Vietnam in the late 1880s and is believed to be derived from a classic French soup, pot au feu. The Vietnamese took influences from both Chinese and French cuisines to create this soup. It is traditionally prepared with bone broth, but we have modified it to keep it plant-based and keto.

8 cups vegetable broth

1-inch knob fresh ginger, peeled and chopped

2 tablespoons tamari

3 cups shredded fresh spinach

2 cups chopped broccoli

1 cup sliced mushrooms

½ cup chopped carrots

⅓ cup chopped scallions

1 (8-ounce) package shirataki noodles

2 cups shredded cabbage

2 cups mung bean sprouts

Fresh Thai basil leaves, for garnish

Fresh cilantro leaves, for garnish

Fresh mint leaves, for garnish

1 lime, cut into 8 wedges, for garnish

1. In a large stockpot over medium-high heat, bring the vegetable broth to a simmer with the ginger and tamari.

2. Once the broth is hot, add the spinach, broccoli, mushrooms, carrots, and scallions, and simmer for a few minutes, just until the vegetables start to become tender.

3. Stir in the shirataki noodles, then remove the pot from the heat and divide the soup among serving bowls.

4. Top each bowl with cabbage, sprouts, basil, cilantro, mint, and a lime wedge.

SUBSTITUTION TIP: *The shirataki noodles can be swapped for another variety. Try mung bean noodles for a thick texture, or zucchini noodles for a light flavor and an extra portion of vegetables.*

Per Serving: Calories: 47; Total fat: <1g; Carbohydrates: 10g; Fiber: 3g; Net carbs: 7g; Protein: 3g

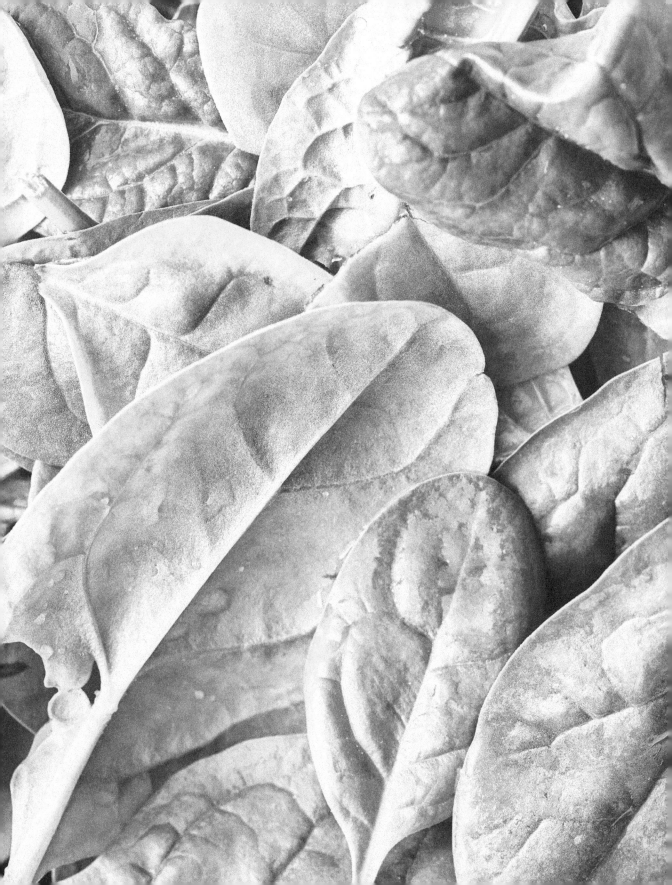

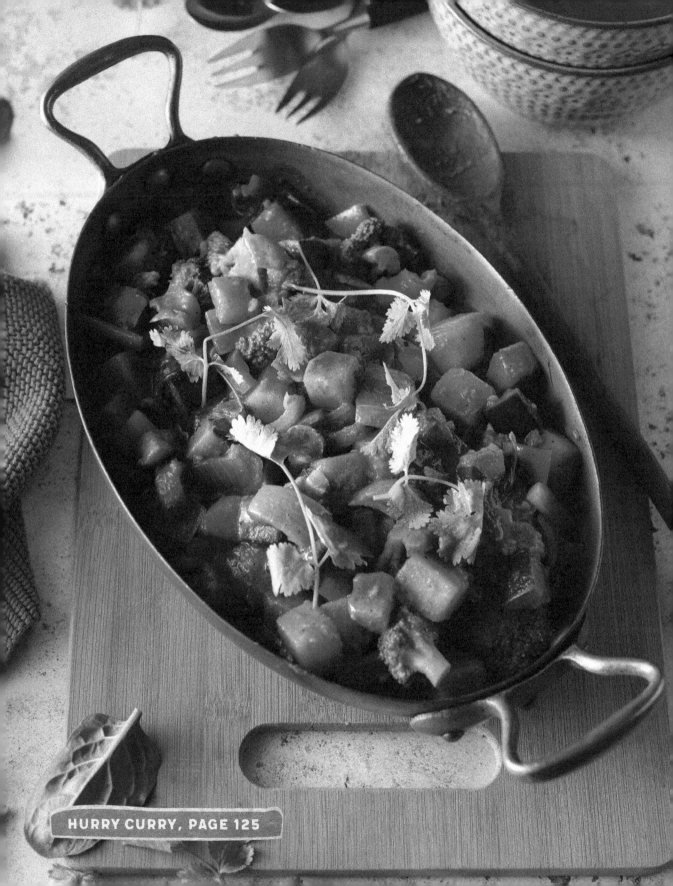

HURRY CURRY, PAGE 125

MAIN DISHES

To curb cravings and stay on track with your macros, it's important to consume nourishing, satisfying meals at lunch and dinner. Equally as crucial is having a variety of flavors and textures to avoid boredom. We've compiled 13 dishes that are sure to tantalize your taste buds every day of the week. Included are some classic food favorites that you may be surprised to learn can easily be made vegan keto. Dive in and pamper your body, baby!

HEARTS OF PALM CAKES

SERVES 4 · PREP TIME: 5 MINUTES · COOK TIME: 10 MINUTES

These are a real crowd pleaser and tough to distinguish from traditional crab cakes. Hearts of palm are very low in both cholesterol and calories and are a good source of protein, fiber; vitamins A, B3, B6, C, and E; and several important minerals such as calcium, potassium, and zinc. When shredded, they resemble crab meat, so they are great for creating these cakes.

FOR THE CAKES

4 cups drained and shredded hearts of palm

2 diced shallots

1 celery stalk, diced

2 tablespoons chopped fresh dill

3 tablespoons vegan mayo

¼ cup seaweed flakes

1 tablespoon Old Bay seasoning

1 tablespoon Dijon mustard

1 tablespoon apple cider vinegar

Sea salt

Freshly ground black pepper

1 cup almond flour

¼ cup coconut oil

FOR THE SAUCE

½ cup Vegan "Sour Cream" (page 46)

4 tablespoons capers

2 tablespoons chopped fresh dill

Juice of ½ lemon, plus 1 lemon cut into 4 wedges, for serving

TO MAKE THE CAKES

1. In a large mixing bowl, combine the hearts of palm, shallots, celery, and dill.
2. Add the vegan mayo, seaweed flakes, Old Bay seasoning, mustard, and apple cider vinegar. Season with salt and pepper. Stir until the ingredients are well combined.
3. Line a plate with paper towels. Set aside. Pour the almond flour into a wide, shallow dish.

4. Divide the mixture into fourths, and use your hands to shape each portion into a small patty. Roll each patty in the almond flour until well coated.

5. In a medium skillet over medium heat, heat the oil.

6. Once the oil is hot, place two cakes in the skillet. Cook until the cakes become golden and toasty on the bottom, about 4 minutes, then flip the cakes and cook for a further 4 minutes.

7. Transfer the cakes to the paper towel-lined plate to absorb excess oil. Repeat step 6 until all the cakes are cooked.

TO MAKE THE SAUCE

To make the sauce, in a high-powered blender, blend together the "sour cream," capers, dill, and lemon juice. Serve the cakes with the sauce and lemon wedges.

COOKING TIP: *For faster preparation, the cakes can be baked instead of pan-fried. Arrange them on a nonstick baking sheet and bake at 350°F for 15 minutes on each side until golden brown.*

Per Serving: Calories: 516; Total fat: 45g; Carbohydrates: 23g; Fiber: 10g; Net carbs: 13g; Protein: 15g

SMOKED SHIITAKE THAI LETTUCE CUPS

SERVES 4 · PREP TIME: 10 MINUTES · COOK TIME: 10 MINUTES

This dish is mostly raw and loaded with vitamins and minerals from the shiitake mushrooms, which boost your immune system, lower cholesterol, and fight cancer. The net carbs here equal 21 grams, so keep this in mind as you plan your meals for the day.

2 tablespoons sesame oil

4 cups thinly sliced shiitake mushrooms

⅓ cup liquid aminos

⅓ cup monk fruit sweetener

3 tablespoons liquid smoke

1 teaspoon paprika

1 teaspoon ground cumin

2 heads butter lettuce, separated into leaves

1 cup shredded carrots

1 cup shredded purple cabbage

1 cup thinly sliced green bell peppers

1 cup sprouts

¼ cup chopped fresh mint

¼ cup chopped fresh cilantro

¼ cup chopped fresh Thai basil

2 tablespoons black sesame seeds

¼ cup Thai-Style Peanut Sauce (page 44)

1. In a medium skillet on medium heat, warm the sesame oil.
2. Add the mushrooms to the skillet and stir until they start to sweat and release a little water.
3. Add the aminos, monk fruit sweetener, liquid smoke, paprika, and cumin, and cook, stirring occasionally to prevent sticking.

4. Once the mushrooms have absorbed most of the liquid and are caramelized, remove the skillet from the heat and set aside.

5. To assemble the lettuce cups, place a small portion of mushrooms in the bottom of each lettuce leaf.

6. Top with the carrots, cabbage, bell pepper, sprouts, mint, cilantro, and basil. Drizzle with peanut sauce and sprinkle with the black sesame seeds before serving.

SUBSTITUTION TIP: *If you're having a hard time finding shiitake mushrooms, you can easily replace them with baby portobello mushrooms. The flavor profile of shiitake is unique and portobello mushrooms absorb more of the liquid smoke flavor, so choose what works best for you.*

Per Serving: Calories: 250; Total fat: 15g; Carbohydrates: 28g; Fiber: 7g; Net carbs: 21g; Protein: 8g

GARLIC FRIED CAULIFLOWER RICE

SERVES 4 · PREP TIME: 10 MINUTES · COOK TIME: 20 MINUTES

Fried rice is not just a dish for elaborate nights at the hibachi house. This "rice" dish is a party for your mouth that won't ruin your keto status and will keep you healthy with all the nutrients contained in each and every ingredient. You'll be back for more, guaranteed.

1 (14-ounce) block sprouted tofu

4 tablespoons nutritional yeast

2 tablespoons tahini

1 teaspoon kala namak salt

1 teaspoon turmeric powder

1 tablespoon sesame oil

1 shallot, chopped

2 garlic cloves, chopped

1 tablespoon ground ginger

1 cup chopped carrots

1 cup peas

6 cups cauliflower rice

½ cup chopped scallions, plus more for garnish

¼ cup tamari, plus more for drizzling

1. Drain the tofu, pressing it with a paper towel to absorb as much water as possible.
2. In a medium mixing bowl, crumble the tofu and mix it with the nutritional yeast, tahini, turmeric, and kala namak to create an egg-like texture.
3. In a large skillet over medium heat, heat the sesame oil and add the shallot, garlic, and ginger, and cook, stirring regularly to prevent burning, until fragrant, about 3 minutes.
4. Add the carrots and peas and cook until the carrots become slightly tender, about 5 minutes.

5. Add the tofu "eggs" to the skillet and toss. Allow the tofu to toast up slightly on each side.

6. Add the cauliflower rice, scallions, and tamari and stir thoroughly to mix all the flavors.

7. Cook for 5 minutes to allow the flavors to meld and any excess liquid to cook off.

8. Remove from the heat, drizzle with a splash of tamari, and garnish with chopped scallions.

MAKE-AHEAD TIP: *This is a great dish for entertaining. You can make this in advance and spoon the finished Garlic Fried Cauliflower Rice into a casserole dish and store covered in your refrigerator until your party. To serve simply pop in the oven at 350°F for 20 minutes to bring it up to temperature and serve.*

Per Serving: Calories: 288; Total fat: 13g; Carbohydrates: 26g; Fiber: 9g; Net carbs: 17g; Protein: 23g

BUDDHA BOWL

We are big fans of food bowls, especially because they are an easy go-to for a fast meal. We have added edamame to make this dish rich in protein, fiber, antioxidants, and vitamin K. This Buddha Bowl is so satisfying and nutritionally dense, you'll have no choice but to become enlightened.

Nonstick coconut oil cooking spray

2 cups cubed butternut squash

⅓ cup coconut oil

Sea salt

Freshly ground black pepper

1 zucchini, spiralized or cut into noodles

1 cup chopped broccoli

½ cup edamame

⅓ cup sliced radishes

⅓ cup black olives

1 avocado, peeled, pitted, and sliced

1 tablespoon Tahini Goddess dressing (page 49)

Sesame seeds, for serving

1. Preheat the oven to 350°F. Grease a baking sheet with cooking spray and set aside.

2. In a large mixing bowl, toss the butternut squash in the coconut oil. Season with salt and pepper.

3. Arrange the squash on the prepared baking sheet and bake for 20 minutes until the squash is tender.

4. Remove the squash from the oven and place in the bottom of the serving bowl.

5. Top with the zucchini spirals, broccoli, edamame, radishes, olives, and avocado.

6. Garnish with the dressing and sprinkle with sesame seeds.

SUBSTITUTION TIP: *This dish is very flexible in terms of ingredients, which makes it a great repeat meal. Just switch up some of the elements to keep things interesting. For instance, swapping the tahini dressing for a different sauce makes the bowl taste completely different.*

Per Serving: Calories: 334; Total fat: 28g; Carbohydrates: 21g; Fiber: 8g; Net carbs: 13g; Protein: 6g

HURRY CURRY

Aptly named, this curry cooks up in a jiffy. In addition to their fragrance and bold taste, the spices also play a role in fighting disease. Curry powder is very powerful at reducing inflammation, fighting cancer, aiding digestion, and combating Alzheimer's.

1 tablespoon coconut oil

1 yellow onion, diced

2 tablespoons grated fresh ginger

2 garlic cloves, minced

3 tablespoons curry powder

1 tablespoon ground cumin

1 tablespoon tomato paste

2 cups chopped butternut squash

1 cup chopped broccoli

1 cup chopped red bell pepper

1 cup chopped eggplant

1 (4-ounce) can coconut cream

⅓ cup vegetable broth

4 cups fresh spinach

1 tablespoon chopped cilantro or Thai basil, for garnish

1. Heat the coconut oil in a large stockpot over medium-high heat.
2. Add the onion, ginger, and garlic to the pot. Cook until the onions become translucent and fragrant, about 3 minutes.
3. Stir in the curry powder, cumin, and tomato paste.
4. Add the squash, broccoli, bell pepper, and eggplant and stir a few times to coat the vegetables with the spices.
5. Stir in the coconut cream and vegetable broth.
6. Reduce the heat to low and simmer for 25 to 30 minutes to allow the curry to become thick and rich.
7. Remove the pot from the heat, add the spinach and cover the pot for a few minutes to let the spinach wilt.
8. Serve in bowls garnished with the cilantro or Thai basil.

INGREDIENT TIP: *Since the spices in this dish are highly anti-inflammatory, this is a great go-to when you're feeling worn down and want to give your immune system a boost.*

Per Serving: Calories: 133; Total fat: 8g; Carbohydrates: 17g; Fiber: 5g; Net carbs: 12g; Protein: 3g

KETO MARGHERIT-O PIZZA

SERVES 4 · PREP TIME: 10 MINUTES · COOK TIME: 25 MINUTES

Pizza is a major food group, right? We couldn't leave it out of our vegan keto cookbook. We have adapted the classic margherita by using a keto-friendly crust and swapping out the dairy cheese for a plant-based alternative.

1 cup lukewarm water

½ cup plus 2 tablespoons coconut flour

2 tablespoons ground psyllium husk

¼ teaspoon sea salt

1 tablespoon cold-pressed olive oil

¼ cup tomato sauce

¼ cup vegan mozzarella

¼ cup sliced mushrooms

¼ cup sliced olives

¼ cup fresh basil leaves, for garnish

1 teaspoon red pepper flakes, for garnish

1. Preheat the oven to 420°F. Prepare two pieces of parchment paper on a work surface. If you don't have parchment paper, use wax paper.
2. In a large mixing bowl, combine the water, coconut flour, psyllium husk, salt, and olive oil, and knead together to form the dough. If it's breaking apart, add more water a tablespoon at a time until the dough sticks together.
3. Set aside and allow the dough to rest for 10 minutes.
4. Turn the dough out onto one piece of parchment paper. Cover with the second piece and roll the dough out into a crust. A thinner crust will create a crisper texture.

5. Peel off the top layer of parchment paper. Leave the bottom piece of parchment paper intact to help slide the crust onto a baking sheet. Bake the crust for 15 minutes.

6. Remove the crust from the oven and top it with the tomato sauce, vegan mozzarella, mushrooms, and olives.

7. Return the pizza to the oven for a further 5 to 7 minutes until the cheese starts to toast and bubble.

8. Allow the pizza to cool for 10 minutes before cutting. Cut with a rolling pizza slicer and serve garnished with the basil and red pepper flakes.

MAKE-AHEAD TIP: *For fast and easy mid-week meal prep, prepare the dough in advance and store it in the freezer. To make it extra convenient, use a rolling pin to shape the dough into a crust and then place between pieces of parchment paper before putting it in the freezer.*

Per Serving: Calories: 159; Total fat: 8g; Carbohydrates: 19g; Fiber: 11g; Net carbs: 8g; Protein: 3g

GINGER-LIME VEGGIE STIR FRY

SERVES 4 · PREP TIME: 10 MINUTES · COOK TIME: 15 MINUTES

Everyone loves an epic stir fry. We made sure to include ginger because of its role in reducing inflammation. This dish is so fragrant, your neighbors will be jealous! With all the vegetables we have used here, you are bound to get in your recommended daily requirement of vitamins. And what a deliciously satisfying way to do it.

3 tablespoons coconut oil

⅓ cup minced scallions, plus more for serving

3 garlic cloves, chopped

1-inch knob ginger root, peeled and grated

½ cup diced butternut squash

½ cup diced celery

½ cup peas

½ cup ribbon-sliced red cabbage

¼ cup tamari, plus more for serving

1 tablespoon sesame oil

Juice of 1 lime, divided

4 cups cauliflower rice

1 teaspoon chili oil

1. In a large skillet on medium heat, heat the coconut oil.
2. When the oil is warm, add the scallions and sauté until translucent, about 3 minutes.
3. Add the garlic and ginger, and cook, stirring often, until fragrant.
4. Stir in the squash, celery, peas, cabbage, tamari, sesame oil, and half the lime juice.
5. Stir-fry until the vegetables become slightly tender, about 10 minutes.
6. Add the cauliflower rice and remaining lime juice and cook for a further 5 minutes.
7. Remove from the heat and garnish with another splash of tamari, some chopped scallions, and the chili oil.

MAKE-AHEAD TIP: *This is a great make-ahead meal because it keeps in the refrigerator for up to 1 week. Store it in an airtight container in the refrigerator and reheat on the stovetop in a covered saucepan.*

Per Serving: Calories: 198; Total fat: 15g; Carbohydrates: 13g; Fiber: 4g; Net carbs: 9g; Protein: 6g

GOOD SHEPHERD'S PIE

SERVES 4 · PREP TIME: 15 MINUTES · COOK TIME: 50 MINUTES

Shepherd's pie is usually loaded with animal products and carbs, so we've lightened things up to keep it vegan. Plus, we substituted the traditional mashed potato topping with a nutritious, low-carb cauliflower mash. We're confident you won't miss a thing. The net carbs here equal 23 grams, so keep this in mind as you plan your meals for the day.

FOR THE MASHED TOPPING

1 head cauliflower, coarsely chopped

Sea salt

¼ cup cold-pressed olive oil

⅓ cup tahini

White pepper

FOR THE FILLING

Nonstick cooking spray

3 tablespoons cold-pressed olive oil, plus more for drizzling

1 yellow onion, chopped

1 shallot, chopped

2 garlic cloves, chopped

2 tablespoons white pepper

2 teaspoons onion powder

1 teaspoon fennel seeds

1 teaspoon ground coriander

1 teaspoon ground cumin

½ cup dry Marsala wine

5 cups chopped mushrooms

1 cup peas

½ cup chopped carrots

½ cup chopped celery

½ cup chopped walnuts

½ cup nutritional yeast

3 cups mushroom broth

1 thyme sprig

1 rosemary sprig, plus more, chopped, for garnish

3 cups fresh spinach

TO MAKE THE MASHED TOPPING

1. Preheat the oven to 375°F.
2. Bring a large pot of water to a boil over high heat. Add the cauliflower and cook for about 12 minutes or until tender.

CONTINUED

3. When cooked, the cauliflower should be so tender that it falls apart easily with a fork. Strain it and return it to the pot.

4. Add the olive oil and tahini and season with salt and white pepper. Mash with a potato masher, or for a creamier finish, whip with an immersion blender. Set aside.

TO MAKE THE FILLING

1. While the cauliflower is cooking, Grease a 9-by-13-inch casserole dish with cooking spray.

2. In a large skillet over medium heat, warm the oil.

3. Add the onion, shallot, and garlic, white pepper, onion powder, fennel, coriander, and cumin to the skillet. Cook until the onions become tender and the spices are fragrant, about 5 minutes.

4. Pour in the Marsala wine to deglaze the pan. Allow the wine to cook off partially, 3 to 4 minutes.

5. Add the mushrooms, peas, carrots, celery, walnuts, and nutritional yeast, and stir to coat the vegetables in the spices.

6. Add the mushroom broth, plus the thyme and rosemary sprigs and simmer for about 20 minutes, until the sauce thickens and reduces.

TO ASSEMBLE THE PIE

1. Arrange the vegetable mixture in an even layer in the prepared casserole dish.

2. Lay the spinach over the vegetables.

3. Top with the cauliflower mash, spreading it evenly to completely cover the spinach layer.

4. Top with a drizzle of olive oil and a sprinkle of rosemary and place in the oven to bake for 25 minutes.

5. Remove from the oven after the top starts to toast. Allow to cool for 10 minutes before serving. To serve, cut into even-sized squares and plate.

INGREDIENT TIP: *Dry Marsala wine is a great flavor-boosting component that can intensify the savory flavor of other ingredients. You'll find it in most markets and liquor stores.*

Per Serving: Calories: 615; Total fat: 46g; Carbohydrates: 37g; Fiber: 14g; Net carbs: 23g; Protein: 24g

SHIRATAKI NOODLES CARBONARA

SERVES 4 · PREP TIME: 5 MINUTES · COOK TIME: 15 MINUTES

This now-classic pasta originated during the American occupation of Rome in 1944, with local chefs using the available Army rations of eggs, bacon, and cheese. We've omitted the cheese and egg, but not the flavor. You'll find the nutritional yeast and the mushrooms give this dish so much substance and savoriness that you may never want to cook it any other way.

1 (8-ounce) package shirataki noodles

4 tablespoons cold-pressed olive oil

½ yellow onion, chopped

1 cup sliced mushrooms

4 garlic cloves, chopped

1½ cups Vegan "Sour Cream" (page 46)

¼ cup nutritional yeast, plus more for serving

½ cup dry white wine

½ cup peas

Freshly ground black pepper

⅓ cup Coconut "Bacon" (see page 98)

¼ cup fresh basil, for garnish

1. Cook the noodles according to the package instructions, and set aside.

2. In a large skillet over medium-high heat, heat the olive oil.

3. Add the onion, mushrooms, and garlic, stirring regularly to prevent burning.

4. Add the "sour cream," nutritional yeast, and white wine, and cook, stirring often, until the wine cooks off and the sauce reduces, about 5 minutes.

5. Add the peas and sauté for 3 minutes until they start to become tender.

6. Taste the sauce and season with pepper to taste.

7. Add the cooked noodles to the skillet, stirring often and allowing them to soak up the sauce for about 3 minutes.

8. Remove from the heat and plate the noodles. Top with the coconut "bacon," basil, more pepper, and a dusting of nutritional yeast.

INGREDIENT TIP: *To mix up the texture of this dish, swap out the shirataki noodles for other types of keto-friendly, plant-based noodles, like those made from zucchini, hearts of palm, or mung bean.*

Per Serving: Calories: 530; Total fat: 46g; Carbohydrates: 23g; Fiber: 8g; Net carbs: 15g; Protein: 19g

WARMING SPICED CHILI

Many people assume that chili has to be loaded with meat and carbs in order to taste good. Surprise! This chili is entirely plant-based and low-carb, yet just as filling and satisfying as traditional chili. Take it to the next Super Bowl party to make everyone a fan.

4 tablespoons cold-pressed olive oil

1 yellow onion, chopped

4 tablespoons chili powder

1 teaspoon ground cumin

1 teaspoon dried oregano

1 teaspoon ground allspice

½ teaspoon ground cinnamon

1 teaspoon ground coriander

2 thyme sprigs

1 can black soybeans, rinsed and drained

½ cup chopped walnuts

¼ cup hemp seeds

2 cups vegetable broth

1 (8-ounce) can chunky stewed tomatoes

3 tablespoons tomato paste

2 cups chopped fresh kale

½ cup chopped scallions, for garnish

Cayenne pepper (optional)

1. In a large stockpot over medium heat, heat the olive oil.
2. Add the onion, chili powder, cumin, oregano, allspice, cinnamon, coriander, and thyme. Cook, stirring regularly, until the onion is tender, about 5 minutes.
3. Add the soybeans, walnuts, hemp seeds, vegetable broth, stewed tomatoes, and tomato paste. Reduce the heat to low and simmer for 45 minutes to allow the chili to thicken and the flavors to meld.
4. Stir in the kale and simmer for 4 more minutes.
5. Remove the chili from the heat and divide equally among small serving bowls.
6. Garnish with the scallions and some cayenne pepper if you want to add a little heat.

MAKE-AHEAD TIP: *For easy meal prep throughout the winter and sports party seasons, make a double batch and store the second half in a freezer-safe container in the freezer. When you're ready, warm it up on the stove or in a microwave.*

Per Serving: Calories: 366; Total fat: 31g; Carbohydrates: 20g; Fiber: 9g; Net carbs: 11g; Protein: 10g

CAULIFLOWER-STUFFED GREEN PEPPERS

SERVES 4 · PREP TIME: 10 MINUTES · COOK TIME: 1 HOUR

One of the best dishes Nicole's mom used to make was stuffed peppers. We are extremely excited to bring you this vegan keto version. The walnuts are known as a good-cancer fighting food, and they also provide brain-healthy fats while adding a fun texture to this dish.

Nonstick cooking spray

5 cups cauliflower rice

4 tablespoons coconut oil, divided

1 tablespoon ground cumin

1 bay leaf

1 teaspoon fennel

1 teaspoon red pepper flakes

3 tablespoons Italian seasoning

½ yellow onion, chopped

3 garlic cloves, chopped

½ cup dry Marsala wine

1 cup coarsely chopped raw walnuts

4 green bell peppers, tops cut off and seeds removed

⅓ cup tomato paste

1 cup vegetable broth

⅓ cup hemp hearts

2 cups chopped fresh spinach

1 cup shredded vegan mozzarella

1. Preheat the oven to 400°F. Grease a medium baking dish with cooking spray.
2. In a medium mixing bowl, coat the cauliflower rice in 2 tablespoons of coconut oil.
3. In a large skillet over medium heat, heat the remaining 2 tablespoons of coconut oil and add the cumin, bay leaf, fennel, red pepper flakes, and Italian seasoning. Add the walnuts to the pan, allowing them to toast on each side for about 3 to 4 minutes. While the nuts are toasting, add the onions and garlic to the skillet.
4. Cook for 3 minutes, stirring occasionally. Once the onions become translucent, deglaze the skillet by pouring in the Marsala wine and then stirring and scraping the bottom of the skillet.

5. Add the tomato paste and vegetable broth, stir, then add the cauliflower and hemp hearts, making sure to coat them thoroughly with the sauce.

6. Arrange the bell peppers in the prepared baking dish.

7. Remove the cauliflower mixture from the heat and stir in the spinach to wilt. Carefully spoon the rice mixture into the hollows of the bell peppers, stuffing them generously. Top with the shredded mozzarella and bake for 35 to 40 minutes, until the bell peppers start to toast and the cheese is melted. Allow to cool before serving, as the temperature inside the peppers can be extremely hot.

8. Serve in shallow bowls, because when you cut into the peppers, a lot of juice will flow out.

LEFTOVERS TIP: *This dish tastes even better the day after preparing it, which makes for delicious leftovers. Reheat your leftover peppers in the oven for a quick mid-week meal.*

Per Serving: Calories: 527; Total fat: 42g; Carbohydrates: 29g; Fiber: 12g; Net carbs: 17g; Protein: 18g

RAINBOW KEBABS

SERVES 4 · PREP TIME: 15 MINUTES ·
COOK TIME: 10 MINUTES, PLUS AT LEAST 30 MINUTES TO MARINATE

Even though neither one of us grew up vegan, our families have always had a fondness for vegetables. Summertime meant poolside grill-outs with veggie-rainbow kebabs on the menu. (Thank you, Mom.) You will need skewers for this recipe. If using bamboo skewers, soak them in water for 1 hour before using to prevent burning.

Juice of 3 limes

⅓ cup tamari

Coconut oil

¼ cup monk fruit sweetener

1 tablespoon Montreal steak seasoning

12 to 15 mushrooms

3 bell peppers variety of colors, cut into bite-size pieces

1 red onion, cut into bite-size pieces

1 zucchini, cut into bite-size pieces

½ pound cherry tomatoes

Nonstick cooking spray

¼ cup Thai-Style Peanut Sauce (page 44)

1. Preheat the grill to medium. If cooking indoors, preheat the oven to 375°F.
2. In a medium mixing bowl, make the marinade by combining the lime juice, tamari, coconut oil, monk fruit sweetener, and Montreal steak seasoning.
3. Add the mushrooms to the bowl and let them marinate for at least 30 minutes and up to overnight for amazing results.
4. Build the skewers by spearing each piece of vegetable through its center and sliding it down the skewer, alternating colors to create a rainbow effect. Leave an inch unfilled on both ends for easier handling.
5. Drizzle the skewers with some of the remaining marinade.

6. Coat the grill with cooking spray. Cook the skewers for 5 to 7 minutes, then rotate them and drizzle with the remaining marinade before cooking for a further 5 minutes. If preparing in the oven, cook on each side for 10 minutes, coating with the marinade halfway through. Turn the oven to broil at the end to create a barbecue-like char, watching carefully to prevent burning.

7. When the vegetables are tender and slightly charred around the edges, remove them from the heat.

8. Drizzle them with the peanut sauce and serve.

LEFTOVERS TIP: *These veggies can be reheated in the microwave and enjoyed right off the stick. You can also turn them into a food bowl by mixing them with some cauliflower rice.*

Per Serving: Calories: 147; Total fat: 6g; Carbohydrates: 18g; Fiber: 5g; Net carbs: 13g; Protein: 9g

CAULIFLOWER TACOS

SERVES 2 · PREP TIME: 20 MINUTES · COOK TIME: 40 MINUTES

Finally, a vegan keto solution for Taco Tuesday! Cauliflower is rich in fiber, which can aid in weight loss. It's also rich in choline, which is essential for learning and memory retention. The net carbs here equal 32 grams, so keep this in mind as you plan your meals for the day.

FOR THE TORTILLAS

1 cup almond flour

½ cup warm water

3 tablespoons ground psyllium husk

½ tablespoon coconut oil

⅛ teaspoon sea salt

1 tablespoon coconut oil, for cooking the tortillas

FOR THE TACOS

1 tablespoon coconut oil

4 cups chopped cauliflower

4 tablespoons taco seasoning

1 cup pico de gallo (fresh, mild, chunky salsa)

1 avocado, peeled, pitted, and sliced

¼ cup chopped fresh cilantro

1 tablespoon Vegan "Sour Cream" (page 46)

1 lime, cut into wedges

TO MAKE THE TORTILLAS

1. In a medium mixing bowl, combine the almond flour, water, psyllium husk, coconut oil, and salt. Using your hands, knead the ingredients together, adding small sprinkles of extra water if necessary, until you've formed a smooth dough. Set aside to rest for up to 10 minutes.

2. Prepare two pieces of pre-greased parchment paper. If you don't have parchment paper, use wax paper.

3. Separate the dough into 4 ball-shaped pieces. Place one dough ball between the two pieces of parchment paper and roll it out until thin.

4. In a medium skillet over medium-high heat, heat the coconut oil.

5. Place a tortilla in the skillet and toast on one side for 3 minutes before flipping and toasting on the opposite side.

6. Remove the tortilla from the heat and set aside in a basket or cover with a towel to keep warm while you repeat step 5 to make the remaining tortillas.

TO MAKE THE TACOS

1. In a medium skillet, heat the coconut oil and carefully drop in the cauliflower. Add the taco seasoning and stir to coat the cauliflower. Sauté until the cauliflower is tender, about 12 minutes. Remove from the heat and set aside.

2. To build the tacos, fill each tortilla with one-quarter of the cauliflower mixture, pico de gallo, avocado, cilantro, and "sour cream." Garnish with a wedge of fresh lime and serve.

INGREDIENT TIP: *Spruce up this dish with flavorful toppings to add variety and extra nutrition. For a probiotic boost, top the tacos with your favorite sauerkraut or kimchi.*

Per Serving: Calories: 832; Total fat: 62g; Carbohydrates: 63g; Fiber: 31g; Net carbs: 32g; Protein: 21g

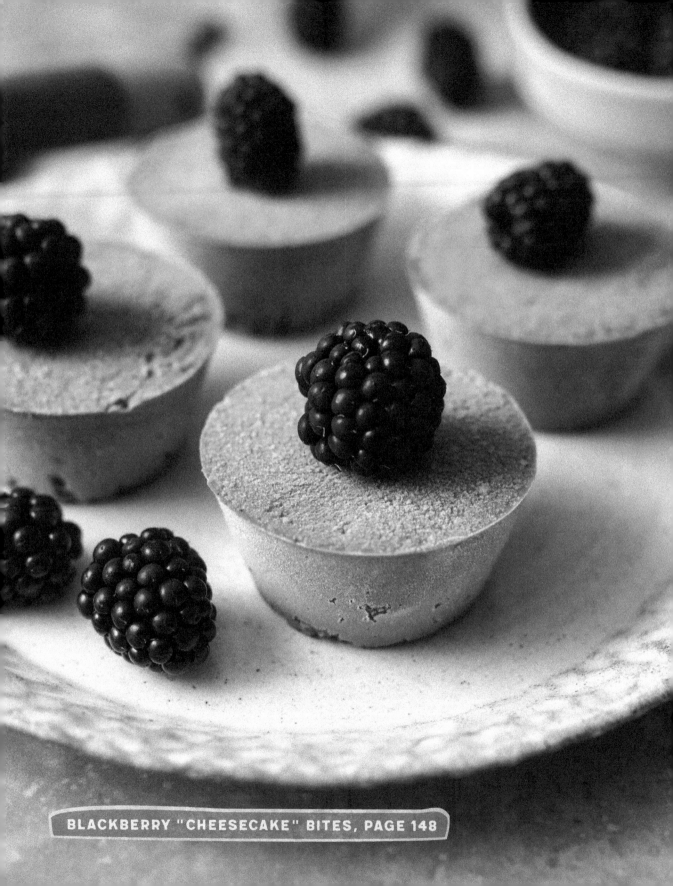

BLACKBERRY "CHEESECAKE" BITES, PAGE 148

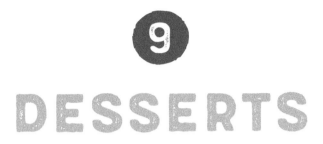

DESSERTS

This might be the most important part of the cookbook, because dessert is very important. If you skipped directly to this chapter, we don't blame you. Just because you're counting your carbs and avoiding sugar doesn't mean you can't satisfy your sweet tooth! Here are eight recipes you can indulge in, including several that feature chocolate. You'll also find traditional crowd-pleasers you can whip up to avoid any feeling of missing out on tasty treats. Once you try these treats, you'll be saying, "Sugar who?"

FUDGE POPS

These chocolatey pops zip us right back to warm childhood nights playing with the neighborhood kids on the front lawn while our moms yelled, "Don't run with those pops in your mouth; it's dangerous!"

1 (14-ounce) can full-fat coconut cream

3 avocados, peeled, pitted, and chopped

⅓ cup cacao powder

5 or 6 drops liquid stevia

⅓ cup freshly grated orange zest

Sea salt

1. In a high-powered blender, combine the coconut cream with the avocados, cacao powder, and stevia.
2. Whip the mixture in the blender for 5 minutes until it becomes airy.
3. Stir in the orange zest and salt and pour the mixture into popsicle molds.
4. Place the molds in the freezer overnight to set.
5. To serve, run warm water over the popsicle molds to loosen the fudge pops.

COOKING TIP: *To add a crunchy texture, add nuts like cashews, macadamia nuts, and/or walnuts. Loosely chop your choice of nuts and sprinkle them in the bottom of the mold before pouring in the popsicle batter. Freeze and enjoy!*

Per Serving: Calories: 434; Total fat: 40g; Carbohydrates: 21g; Fiber: 12g; Net carbs: 9g; Protein: 4g

LAVENDER ICE CREAM

SERVES 4 · PREP TIME: 5 MINUTES, PLUS 5 HOURS TO FREEZE

Flowers in desserts are beautiful. The lavender in this ice cream is delightful and calming, the coconut cream is full of satisfying fat, and the cashews are loaded with protein. One scoop after a filling meal and you'll be sleeping like a baby.

2 (14-ounce) cans full-fat coconut cream

¾ cup monk fruit sweetener

½ cup raw cashews, soaked in water overnight

¼ cup coconut oil, melted

3 tablespoons dried lavender

1 teaspoon vanilla extract1 teaspoon almond extract

Sea salt

1. Combine all the ingredients in a high-powered blender and blend on high for 5 minutes until the mixture grows in volume by about one-third and becomes fluffy.

2. Pour the mixture into a freezer-safe pan and freeze for 2 hours.

3. Remove the mixture from the freezer and break it into chunks.

4. Transfer the mixture to a food processor and blend until a soft-serve consistency is achieved.

5. Spoon the ice cream into a freezer-safe pan and place back in the freezer to set for 3 hours before serving.

USE IT AGAIN TIP: *This ice cream pairs nicely with Lemon-Poppyseed Cookies (page 146). For an extra impressive presentation, create an ice cream sandwich by placing a generous scoop of ice cream in between two cookies.*

Per Serving: Calories: 571; Total fat: 60g; Carbohydrates: 10g; Fiber: 1g; Net carbs: 9g; Protein: 3g

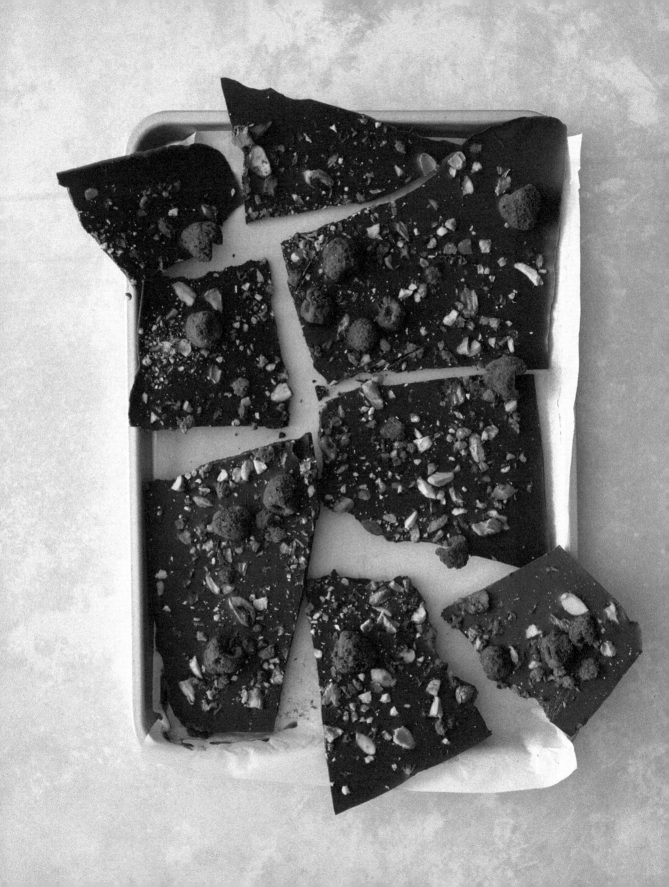

PISTACHIO-RASPBERRY CHOCOLATE BARK

SERVES 4 · PREP TIME: 5 MINUTES

One can accomplish just about anything with some good chocolate. This sweet treat makes a great vegan keto dessert to take to holiday season pot-lucks. The net carbs here equal 27 grams, so keep this in mind as you plan your meals for the day.

Nonstick cooking spray

6 ounces unsweetened dark chocolate

⅓ cup monk fruit sweetener

1 tablespoon coconut oil

¼ cup pistachios, crushed

¼ cup freeze-dried raspberries

Sea salt

1. Line a baking sheet with parchment paper, wax paper, or aluminum foil. Grease it with nonstick spray and set aside.
2. Using a double boiler or a bowl set over a pan of simmering water (the bowl shouldn't touch the water), slowly melt the chocolate.
3. Once the chocolate has melted, stir in the monk fruit sweetener and coconut oil and cook on low for one minute until the ingredients are mixed and chocolate is silky.
4. Pour the chocolate mixture onto the prepared baking sheet. Tap the sheet on the countertop to spread the chocolate out evenly and remove bubbles.
5. Before the chocolate hardens, generously sprinkle it with the pistachios, raspberries, and sea salt.
6. Place the baking sheet in the refrigerator for 2 hours to let the chocolate firm up.
7. Remove the sheet from the refrigerator and break the chocolate into rough chunks. Store in an airtight container in the refrigerator.

MAKE-AHEAD TIP: *Make this chocolate bark ahead of time and store it in the freezer as a perfect go-to when cravings strike.*

Per Serving: Calories: 248; Total fat: 20g; Carbohydrates: 28g; Fiber: 1g; Net carbs: 27g; Protein: 4g

LEMON-POPPYSEED COOKIES

SERVES 4 · PREP TIME: 5 MINUTES · COOK TIME: 10 MINUTES

Sometimes you have a craving for something sweet but don't want your treat to be too decadent. We've got you covered with these sweet little lemon-poppy cookies, which are nice and light. What's more, the poppy seeds contain essential minerals, so you can get away with calling these healthy.

Nonstick cooking spray

1 cup almond butter

¾ cup monk fruit sweetener

4 tablespoons chia seeds

3 tablespoons fresh grated lemon zest

Juice of 1 lemon

1 tablespoon poppy seeds

1. Preheat the oven to 350°F. Grease a baking sheet with cooking spray and set aside.
2. In a large mixing bowl, combine the almond butter with the monk fruit sweetener, chia seeds, lemon zest, lemon juice, and poppy seeds. Mix well, kneading the mixture with your hands.
3. Roll pieces of the dough into cookie-size balls and place them on the prepared baking sheet, spacing them evenly, as some spreading will occur during baking.
4. Bake the cookies for 8 minutes, until golden.
5. Transfer the cookies to a cooling rack.
6. Serve as is or paired with your favorite unsweetened, plant-based milk.

STORAGE TIP: *To keep cookies tender, store them in an airtight container. Layer the cookies with paper towels to absorb excess oil and keep them fresh.*

Per Serving: Calories: 460; Total fat: 39g; Carbohydrates: 21g; Fiber: 12g; Net carbs: 9g; Protein: 13g

COCONUT MACAROONS

SERVES 4 · PREP TIME: 5 MINUTES · COOK TIME: 15 MINUTES

These might as well be called little angel puffs of coconut heaven because that's what they are. The heart-healthy fat and fiber, plus the triple dose of coconut, make this a vegan keto dream.

Nonstick cooking spray

1 cup unsweetened coconut flakes

½ cup coconut milk

⅓ cup monk fruit sweetener

2 tablespoons coconut oil

¼ teaspoon vanilla extract

¼ teaspoon sea salt

1. Preheat the oven to 350°F. Line a baking sheet with parchment paper and grease it with cooking spray. If you don't have parchment paper, use aluminum foil or grease the pan. Set aside.

2. In a high-powered blender, pulse the coconut flakes until they have a meal-like texture.

3. Transfer the coconut to a large mixing bowl and combine it with the coconut milk, monk fruit sweetener, coconut oil, vanilla, and salt.

4. Knead the mixture with your hands to create a dough.

5. Roll pieces of the dough into bite-size balls and place them on the prepared baking sheet.

6. Bake for 15 minutes, checking often to avoid burning. When you see the bottom edges of the macaroons become golden, it's time to remove them from the oven.

7. Transfer the macaroons to a cooling rack and allow them to cool for 20 minutes before serving.

COOKING TIP: *For a more impressive presentation, drizzle the macaroons with melted dark chocolate. Using a double boiler, melt some dark chocolate with 1 teaspoon of coconut oil on low heat. Once the chocolate becomes liquid, drizzle over the macaroons. Place them in the refrigerator to allow the chocolate to set.*

Per Serving: Calories: 212; Total fat: 22g; Carbohydrates: 5g; Fiber: 2g; Net carbs: 3g; Protein: 1g

BLACKBERRY "CHEESECAKE" BITES

SERVES 4 · PREP TIME: 5 MINUTES, PLUS OVERNIGHT TO SOAK AND 1 HOUR 30 MINUTES TO SET

That famous cheesecake restaurant doesn't have a thing on this dessert. These satisfying bites are so much healthier with the fat from the coconut, protein from the almonds, and antioxidants from the blackberries. Not to mention the sugar-free sweetness. It's a one-two-three-four power punch. Who says dessert isn't good for you?

1½ cups almonds, soaked overnight

1 cup blackberries

⅓ cup coconut oil, melted

¼ cup full-fat coconut cream

⅓ cup monk fruit sweetener

¼ cup freshly squeezed lemon juice

1. Prepare a muffin tin by lining the cups with cupcake liners. Set aside.
2. In a high-powered blender, combine the soaked almonds, blackberries, melted coconut oil, coconut cream, monk fruit sweetener, and lemon juice.
3. Blend on high until the mixture is whipped and fluffy.
4. Divide the mixture equally among the muffin cups.
5. Place the muffin tin in the freezer for 90 minutes to allow the cheesecake bites to set.

MAKE-AHEAD TIP: *This dessert works great as a pre-prepared item, particularly for special occasions because you can keep it in the freezer. To thaw, place the bites on the countertop for 1 hour to come to room temperature.*

Per Serving: Calories: 514; Total fat: 48g; Carbohydrates: 18g; Fiber: 9g; Net carbs: 9g; Protein: 12g

CHOCOLATE MOUSSE PIE CUPS

SERVES 6 · PREP TIME: 10 MINUTES, PLUS 1 HOUR 30 MINUTES TO SET

We're suckers for chocolate (in case you didn't already get that). Sure, at first blush the ingredients may seem a little puzzling, but trust us, the taste and texture of this dessert is simply delightful. Not to mention that it contains a ton of heart-healthy fats and omegas.

¾ cup coconut flour

2 flax "eggs" (see page 39)

½ cup coconut oil

4 avocados, peeled, pitted, and chopped

4 tablespoons cacao powder

3 tablespoons monk fruit sweetener

Sea salt

1. Fill the cups of a muffin tin with cupcake liners.
2. In a large mixing bowl, combine the coconut flour, flax "eggs," and coconut oil. Mix thoroughly until you have a workable dough.
3. Scoop the dough a tablespoon at a time into the bottom of the cupcake liners, pressing it firmly to create a crust.
4. Place the muffin tin in the refrigerator for 1 hour to allow the crusts to firm up while you create the pie filling.
5. In a large mixing bowl, combine the avocados, cacao powder, and monk fruit sweetener. Whip with a hand mixer on high until the mixture is well blended and airy.
6. Remove the muffin tin from refrigerator and divide the chocolate mousse mixture equally onto the prepared pie crusts.
7. Place the tin back in the refrigerator to set for 20 to 30 minutes before serving.

SUBSTITUTION TIP: *Omit the crust and serve the mousse by itself for a lighter dessert. Serve in elegant stemmed glassware for an impactful presentation. Sprinkle with berries, coconut flakes, and/or nuts to take it to another level.*

Per Serving: Calories: 439; Total fat: 39g; Carbohydrates: 24g; Fiber: 16g; Net carbs: 8g; Protein: 6g

MEASUREMENT CONVERSIONS

	US STANDARD	US STANDARD (OUNCES)	METRIC (APPROXIMATE)
VOLUME EQUIVALENTS (LIQUID)	2 tablespoons	1 fl. oz.	30 mL
	¼ cup	2 fl. oz.	60 mL
	½ cup	4 fl. oz.	120 mL
	1 cup	8 fl. oz.	240 mL
	1½ cups	12 fl. oz.	355 mL
	2 cups or 1 pint	16 fl. oz.	475 mL
	4 cups or 1 quart	32 fl. oz.	1 L
	1 gallon	128 fl. oz.	4 L
VOLUME EQUIVALENTS (DRY)	⅛ teaspoon		0.5 mL
	¼ teaspoon		1 mL
	½ teaspoon		2 mL
	¾ teaspoon		4 mL
	1 teaspoon		5 mL
	1 tablespoon		15 mL
	¼ cup		59 mL
	⅓ cup		79 mL
	½ cup		118 mL
	⅔ cup		156 mL
	¾ cup		177 mL
	1 cup		235 mL
	2 cups or 1 pint		475 mL
	3 cups		700 mL
	4 cups or 1 quart		1 L
	½ gallon		2 L
	1 gallon		4 L
WEIGHT EQUIVALENTS	½ ounce		15 g
	1 ounce		30 g
	2 ounces		60 g
	4 ounces		115 g
	8 ounces		225 g
	12 ounces		340 g
	16 ounces or 1 pound		455 g

	FAHRENHEIT (F)	CELSIUS (C) (APPROXIMATE)
OVEN TEMPERATURES	250°F	120°C
	300°F	150°C
	325°F	180°C
	375°F	190°C
	400°F	200°C
	425°F	220°C
	450°F	230°C

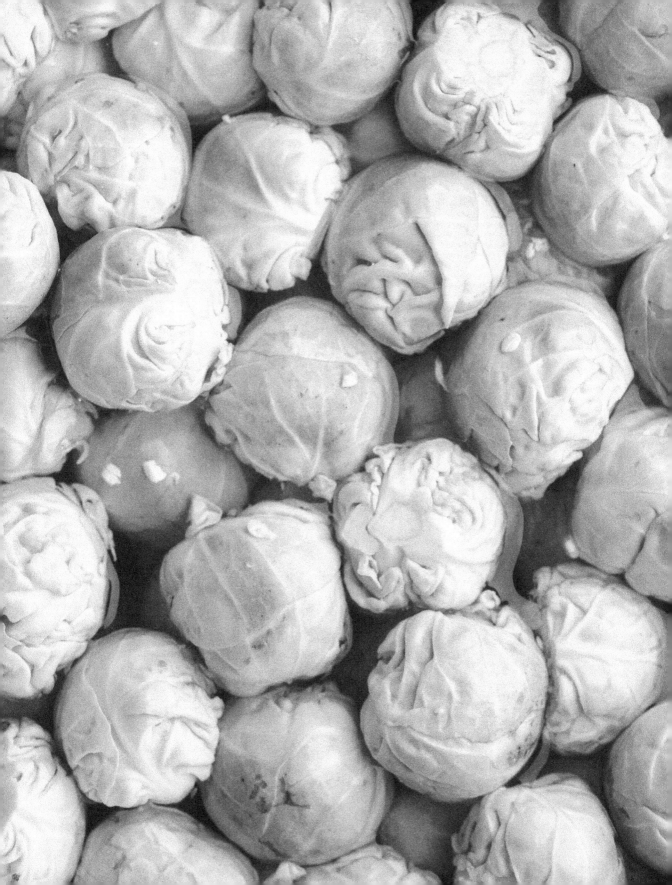

RESOURCES

Brands

Bhu Foods bars

Bragg Live Foods apple cider vinegar and nutritional yeast

BRAMI lupini beans

Bulletproof coffee, XCT Oil, and Brain Octane Oil

Cascadian Farm frozen vegetables

Cave Shake drinks

Cece's Veggie Co. noodles

Chameleon Cold-Brew coffee

ChocZero syrups and chocolates

Chosen Foods oils

Dang Foods bars

Doctor in the Kitchen flax crackers

Earth Balance vegan butter

Eating Evolved chocolate treats

Eden Organic canned beans

Elmhurst 1925 plant-based milk

Foods Alive flax crackers

Four Sigmatic coffee

Gloriously Vegan Noochy Licious nutritional yeast

GT's Living Foods Cocoyo yogurt

Jealous Sweets candy

Lakanto monk fruit products

Lily's Sweets sugar-free chocolate chips and bars

Love Good Fats bars

MatchaBar matcha green tea powder

Melissa's Produce

Miracle Noodles Shirataki noodles

Miyoko's Kitchen butter and cheeses

Navitas Organics superfoods

No Cow bars

NuNaturals syrups

Nutiva oils, proteins, superfoods, spreads and baking products

Omica Organics organic stevia products

Pacific Foods vegetable broth

Palmini low-carb pasta

Pique tea

Pop Zest nutritional yeast

Protes protein chips

Rhythm Superfoods snacks

Ripple dairy-free milk

SeaSnax nori sheets

Smart Sweets gelatin-free gummy candies

Spicely Organics organic herbs and spices

Sunwarrior protein powder

Sweetleaf Stevia liquid stevia

Swerve sweetener

Truvani protein powder

You Are Loved Foods monk fruit sweetener

Books

Fat for Fuel: A Revolutionary Diet to Combat Cancer, Boost Brain Power, and Increase Your Energy, **by Joseph Mercola**

This book does a deep dive into the scientific and medical benefits of keto. It's an in-depth guide on how to optimize health by improving metabolism through a high-fat, low-carb diet.

Genius Foods: Become Smarter, Happier, and More Productive While Protecting Your Brain for Life, **by Max Lugavere and Paul Grewal**

Based on scientific research, this comprehensive guide covers how to improve brain health and achieve peak mental performance through nutrition. The author recommends a low-carbohydrate eating plan to support cognitive health.

Ketotarian: The (Mostly) Plant-Based Plan to Burn Fat, Boost Your Energy, Crush Your Cravings, and Calm Inflammation, **by Will Cole**

A doctor's take on a meat-free keto diet, including his expert advice on how to create a plant-centered, low-carb action plan. Note: recipes featuring eggs and seafood are included.

Superfuel: Ketogenic Keys to Unlock the Secrets of Good Fats, Bad Fats, and Great Health, **by James DiNicolantonio and Joseph Mercola**

Two doctors clarify the compelling benefits of high-fat foods and share detailed advice on the low-carb diet, including vital information on cyclical ketogenic eating.

The Real Food Grocery Guide: Navigate the Grocery Store, Ditch Artificial and Unsafe Ingredients, Bust Nutritional Myths, and Select the Healthiest Foods Possible, **by Maria Marlowe**

A great resource on how to shop for nutritious, high-quality food without getting overwhelmed or confused by labels, marketing terms, and buzz words. Learn how to get the most bang for your buck and the best way to store foods so they last as long as possible.

Vegan Keto, **by Liz MacDowell**

If you're looking for more meals to make, the delicious recipes in Liz's vegan keto cookbook are a fantastic complement to the book in your hands.

Websites and Mobile Applications

Lifesum mobile app
Track your macros by inputting the food items and meals you eat each day, which will keep you on track for ketosis. Plus, this app will remind you to stay hydrated and reach your fitness goals.

MeatFreeKeto.com
Recipes and meal plans developed by Liz MacDowell, author of the Vegan Keto *cookbook. It also features tips and tricks for succeeding with the plant-based, low-carb lifestyle.*

MyFitnessPal website and app
A free online calorie counter and diet plan where you can input recipes and meals to determine detailed nutrition facts and macro ratios.

Nuts.com
Great prices on nuts, seeds, superfood powders, sugar-free chocolate, coffee, tea, and more.

PerfectKeto.com

Online store featuring the brand's products, such as their vegan MCT oils and powders, instant coffee, nut butters, and ketone testing strips. The site also has a blog and podcast with helpful information about the keto lifestyle.

Plan to Eat meal planner website and app

Meal planning program to input and store recipes, plan when to eat them using a visual calendar, and create grocery lists to aid with shopping trips.

Ruled.me

Helpful website about the keto diet that features a calculator and nutrition profile, meal plans, recipes, food lists, and various tips on low-carb living.

TheBigMansWorld.com

A diverse selection of mouthwatering recipes that are mainly vegan and often keto, including desserts, breakfasts, snacks, and meal-prep ideas.

ThriveMarket.com

An impressive online market selling natural products at wholesale prices. This shop mostly features organic brands and has a ketogenic category with an option to narrow down the list to vegan items.

Social media hashtags: #Veganketo and #Ketovegan

Follow these hashtags on social media to get meal inspirations, product recommendations, and tips from other people eating a plant-based, low-carb diet.

REFERENCES

Bough, K.J., Wetherington, J.P., Hassel, B., Paré, J., Gawryluk, J.W., Greene, J.G., Shaw, R., Smith, Y., Geiger, J., and R.J. Dingledine. "Mitochondrial Biogenesis in the Anticonvulsant Mechanism of the Ketogenic Diet." *Annals of Neurology*, 60, no. 2 (2006): 223–35.

Bueno, N., I. de Melo, S. de Oliveira, and T. da Rocha Ataide. "Very-Low-Carbohydrate Ketogenic Diet v. Low-Fat Diet for Long-Term Weight Loss: A Meta-Analysis of Randomised Controlled Trials." *British Journal of Nutrition* (2013).

Cleveland Clinic Health Essentials Podcast, "A Functional Approach to the Keto Diet with Mark Hyman, MD" (transcript), October 3, 2018. my.clevelandclinic.org/podcasts/health-essentials/a-functional-approach-to-the-keto-diet-with-mark-hyman.

Cole, Will. *Ketotarian: The (Mostly) Plant-Based Plan to Burn Fat, Boost Your Energy, Crush Your Cravings, and Calm Inflammation.* New York: Avery, 2018.

DiNicolantonio, James and Joseph Mercola. *Superfuel: Ketogenic Keys to Unlock the Secrets of Good Fats, Bad Fats, and Great Health.* Carlsbad, CA: Hay House, 2018.

Miles, Fayth L., Lloren, Jan Irene C., Haddad, Ella, Siegl, Karen Jaceldo, Knutsen, Synnove, Sabate, Joan, and Gary E. Fraser. "Plasma, Urine, and Adipose Tissue Biomarkers of Dietary Intake Differ Between Vegetarian and Non-Vegetarian Diet Groups in the Adventist Health Study-2." *The Journal of Nutrition*, 149 no. 4 (April 2019).

Gibson, A. A., R. V. Seimon, C. M. Lee, J. Ayre, J. Franklin, T. P. Markovic, et al. "Do Ketogenic Diets Really Suppress Appetite?" (2015).

Intergovernmental Panel on Climate Change, The. Accessed December 7, 2019. https://www.ipcc.ch/.

Kanneganti, T. D. "Inflammatory Bowel Disease and the NLRP3 Inflammasome." *New England Journal of Medicine* (August 2017).

Mac, Lorenz. "The Cyclical Ketogenic Diet: Strategic Carbohydrate Intake for the Keto Athlete." Perfect Keto blog, (September 10, 2018).

Herrero, Mario, Havlík, Peter, Valin, Hugo, Notenbaert, An, Rufino, Mariana C., Thornton, Philip K., Blümmel, Michael, Weiss, Franz, Grace, Delia, and Michael Obersteiner. "Global Livestock: Biomass Use, Production, and GHG." *Proceedings of the National Academy of Sciences* (Dec. 2013).

Masino, S. A., and D. N. Ruskin. "Ketogenic Diets and Pain." *Journal of Child Neurology* 28 no. 8 (August 213):993–1001. doi:10.1177/0883073813487595.

McMacken M, and S. Shah. "A Plant-Based Diet for the Prevention and Treatment of Type 2 Diabetes." *Journal of Geriatric Cardiology* 14 no.5 (May 2017): 342–354.

Mercola, Joseph. *Fat for Fuel: A Revolutionary Diet to Combat Cancer, Boost Brain Power, and Increase Your Energy.* Carlsbad, CA: Hay House, 2017.

Mercola, Joseph. "Ketogenic Diet: A Beginner's Ultimate Guide to Keto." https://articles.mercola.com/ketogenic-diet.aspx.

Moodie, Alison. "Keto Diet for Beginners: Your Complete Guide.". Accessed December 7, 2019. https://www.bulletproof.com/diet/keto/keto-diet-beginners-guide/.

National Health and Nutrition Examination Survey (NHANES) 2009-2010. "What We Eat in America." Accessed August 24, 2019. www.ars.usda.gov/ARSUserFiles/80400530/pdf/0910/Table_1_NIN_GEN_09.pdf.

Nylen, K., Velazquez, J. L., Sayed, V., Gibson, K. M., Burnham, W. M., and O.C. Snead., 3rd (2009). "The Effects of a Ketogenic Diet on ATP Concentrations and the Number of Hippocampal Mitochondria in Aldh5a1(-/-) Mice." *Biochimica et biophysica acta* 1790(3): 208–212. doi:10.1016/j.bbagen.2008.12.005.

Paoli A., and L. Cenci, K.A. Grimaldi. "Effect of Ketogenic Mediterranean Diet with Phytoextracts and Low Carbohydrates/High-Protein Meals on Weight, Cardiovascular Risk Factors, Body Composition and Diet Compliance in Italian Council Employees." *Nutrition Journal* (October 2011).

Paoli A. (2014). "Ketogenic Diet for Obesity: Friend or Foe?" *International Journal of Environmental Research and Public Health*11 no. 2 (Feb. 2014): 2092–2107. doi:10.3390/ijerph110202092.

Hyde, Parker N., Sapper, Teryn N., Crabtree, Christopher D., LaFountain, Richard A., Bowling, Madison L., Buga, Alex, Fell, Brandon, McSwiney, Fionn T., Dickerson, Ryan M., and Vincent J. Miller, "Dietary Carbohydrate Restriction Improves Metabolic Syndrome Independent of Weight Loss." *JCI Insight*, (2019).

Pot, G.K., Battjes, M.C., O. N. Patijn et al. "Nutrition and Lifestyle Intervention in Type 2 Diabetes: Pilot Study in the Netherlands Showing Improved Glucose Control and Reduction in Glucose Lowering Medication." *BMJ Nutrition, Prevention & Health* (2019).

Stern L., Iqbal, N., P. Seshadri, et al. "The Effects of Low-Carbohydrate versus Conventional Weight Loss Diets in Severely Obese Adults: One-Year Follow-up of a Randomized Trial." *Annals of Internal Medicine* (2004).

Volek, J. S., Phinney, S. D., Forsythe, C. E., Quann, E. E., Wood, R. J., Puglisi, M. J., Kraemer, W. J., Bibus,D. M., Fernandez M. L., and R. D. Feinman. "Carbohydrate Restriction Has a More Favorable Impact on the Metabolic Syndrome than a Low Fat Diet." *Lipids* (2009).

Westman, Eric C., Williams, S. Yancy, Jr., Mavropoulos, John C., Marguart, Megan, and Jennifer R. McDuffie. "The Effect of a Low-carbohydrate, Ketogenic Diet Versus a Low-glycemic Index Diet on Glycemic Control in Type 2 Diabetes Mellitus." *Nutrition and Metabolism* (2013).

Yancy W.S., M.K. Olsen, J.R. Guyton, et al. "A Low-Carbohydrate, Ketogenic Diet versus a Low-Fat Diet to Treat Obesity and Hyperlipidemia: A Randomized, Controlled Trial." *Annals of Internal Medicine* (2004).

Youm Y. H., Nguyen, K.Y., Grant, R. W., Goldberg, E. L., Bodogai, M., Kim, D., et al. "The Ketone Metabolite β-hydroxybutyrate Blocks NLRP3 Inflammasome-Mediated Inflammatory Disease." *Nature Medicine* 21 no. 3 (March 2015): 263-9.

INDEX

ACKNOWLEDGMENTS

To both of our families . . . Nicole would like to thank her late southern grandmother, Martha Ann Sills, for sharing the joy of cooking with her as an expression of love. Martha Ann served as Nicole's driving motivation to become plant-based and find ways to help heal and prevent chronic disease in her family lineage for this generation and those to come. Nicole is also grateful to her sister Mindy for embarking on this vegan voyage with her. Whitney sends gratitude to her parents, Marc and Joy, and sister Mary for cheering her on throughout her dietary experiments. Here's to sharing long, healthy lives with our loved ones while creating new family traditions.

We're eternally thankful for our close friends. Special appreciation goes out to our dear friend and vegan author Jason Wrobel for the ongoing inspiration and emotional support during the book writing process (and beyond). It was through Jason that Whitney and Nicole met, so this book literally wouldn't exist without his introduction.

Thank you to Liz MacDowell and Dr. Will Cole for confirming that it's possible to thrive on a keto diet without animal products. And to Dr. Joseph Mercola for advocating for the health benefits of a high-fat, low-carb diet.

Publishing a book has been a dream for both of us. We are deeply grateful that Elizabeth Castoria came to us with the opportunity. Our gratitude also goes out to our editor Carolyn Abate and the whole team at Rockridge Press for guiding us through the process with so much grace.

Whitney would like to thank Andrew Green and Melissa Glazewski for their ongoing encouragement and assistance throughout her personal and professional life. And Nik Tyler for inspiring her to go vegan in 2003 before it was cool . . . who are we kidding? Veganism has always been cool.

Nicole would also like to thank her spiritual teachers and guides for helping her discover self-love and find her life's purpose. Thank you for your light and inspiration, Thich Nhat Hanh, Maya Angelou, Eckhart Tolle, Oprah, Abraham Hicks, Louise Hay, Matt Kahn, Guru Singh, Leslie Kahn, Bali, and the Universe.

And how could we leave out our animal companions Evie, Kashmere, Rez, Bruno, and Basil, who sat by our sides, morning through night, as we completed this book? They're the real MVPs, and the world is a better place thanks to their unconditional love.

ABOUT THE AUTHORS

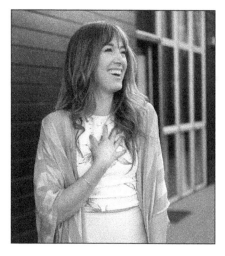

NICOLE DERSEWEH is a vegan chef who comes from a long heritage of family chefs and has a culinary background from Le Cordon Bleu. She is building a worldwide conscious-media empire to inspire vegan newbies with her uplifting and entertaining YouTube channel as one of the cornerstones. You can experience her creations at high-end events and exclusive pop-up dinners in and around the Los Angeles area. Her innovative and delicious plant-based creations consistently impress even the most skeptical critics. Her passion is to share the love, excitement, and compassion of vegan living through decadent dishes that persuade even the most ardent meat-lovers to smile. She could be described as the vegan love child of Rachael Ray and Ellie Kemper. Follow Nicole's journey online @Nicolederseweh on Instagram and YouTube.

WHITNEY LAURITSEN, founder of Eco-Vegan Gal, is a content creator, business coach, and healthy living crusader. With more than 5 million views, her YouTube channels share vegan lifestyle advice, recipes, product reviews, interviews, and inspiration for living in harmony with the body and planet. Whitney is the co-host of "This Might Get Uncomfortable," a podcast she began with her best pal Jason Wrobel. Together they also run the online wellness brand Wellevatr. Whitney is the author of a self-published ebook entitled

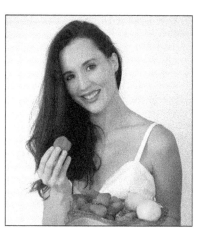

Healthy Organic Vegan on a Budget and has contributed to media outlets such as *VegNews* magazine. She lives in Los Angeles with her vegan Jack Russell Terrier, Evie. Learn more and connect with her at WhitneyLauritsen.com.

CPSIA information can be obtained
at www.ICGtesting.com
Printed in the USA
JSHW032247010821
17309JS00001B/1